SITTING TOGETHER

Also available

SITTING TOGETHER

Essential Skills for Mindfulness-Based Psychotherapy

SUSAN M. POLLAK
THOMAS PEDULLA
RONALD D. SIEGEL

THE GUILFORD PRESS
New York   London

© 2014 The Guilford Press
A Division of Guilford Publications, Inc.
72 Spring Street, New York, NY 10012
www.guilford.com

Printed in the United States of America

This book is printed on acid-free paper.

Last digit is print number: 9 8 7 6 5 4 3 2

The authors have checked with sources believed to be reliable in their efforts to provide information that is complete and generally in accord with the standards of practice
that are accepted at the time of publication. However, in view of the possibility of
human error or changes in behavioral, mental health, or medical sciences, neither the
authors, nor the editor and publisher, nor any other party who has been involved in
the preparation or publication of this work warrants that the information contained
herein is in every respect accurate or complete, and they are not responsible for any
errors or omissions or the results obtained from the use of such information. Readers
are encouraged to confirm the information contained in this book with other sources.

Library of Congress Cataloging-in-Publication Data

Pollak, Susan.
 Sitting together : essential skills for mindfulness-based psychotherapy / by Susan
M. Pollak, Thomas Pedulla, and Ronald D. Siegel.
     pages cm
 Includes bibliographical references and index.
 ISBN 978-1-4625-1398-7 (hard cover : alk. paper)
 1. Mindfulness-based cognitive therapy.   2. Meditation—Therapeutic use.
3. Psychotherapy.   I. Pedulla, Thomas.   II. Siegel, Ronald D.   III. Title.
 RC489.M55P65 2014
 616.89′1425–dc23   2013042212

To our families, teachers, colleagues, patients,
and everyone else with whom we've had
the honor of sitting together

About the Authors

Susan M. Pollak, MTS, EdD, is Clinical Instructor in Psychology at Harvard Medical School, Cambridge Health Alliance, where she has taught and supervised since the mid-1990s. She is President of the Institute for Meditation and Psychotherapy (IMP) and a psychologist in private clinical practice in Cambridge, Massachusetts. A longtime student of meditation and yoga, Dr. Pollak teaches about mindfulness and compassion in psychotherapy and has been integrating the practices of meditation into psychotherapy since the 1980s. Dr. Pollak is the coeditor of *The Cultural Transition* and a contributing author to *Mapping the Moral Domain, Evocative Objects,* and *Mindfulness and Psychotherapy, Second Edition.*

Thomas Pedulla, LICSW, is a clinical social worker and psychotherapist in private practice in Arlington, Massachusetts, where he works with individuals and leads mindfulness-based cognitive therapy groups. A faculty and board member at the IMP since 2007, Mr. Pedulla has also served on the board of the Cambridge Insight Meditation Center and has been a practitioner of meditation in the vipassana tradition since the 1980s. He is a contributing author to *Mindfulness and Psychotherapy, Second Edition.*

Ronald D. Siegel, PsyD, is Assistant Clinical Professor of Psychology at Harvard Medical School, Cambridge Health Alliance, where he has taught since the early 1980s. He is a longtime student of mindfulness meditation and is a faculty and board member at the IMP. Dr. Siegel teaches internationally about mindfulness and psychotherapy and mind–body treatment, while maintaining a private clinical practice in Lincoln, Massachusetts. He is the author of *The Mindfulness Solution: Everyday Practices for Everyday Problems,* coauthor of *Back Sense: A Revolutionary Approach to Halting the Cycle of Chronic Back Pain,* and coeditor of *Wisdom and Compassion in Psychotherapy* and of *Mindfulness and Psychotherapy, Second Edition.*

Preface

> The best of modern therapy is much like a process of shared
> meditation, where therapist and client sit together, learning to
> pay close attention to those aspects and dimensions of the self
> that the client may be unable to touch on his or her own.
> —JACK KORNFIELD (1993, p. 244)

Along with our colleagues at the Institute for Meditation
and Psychotherapy, the three of us have been sitting together, talking
together, and teaching together about the interface between meditation
and psychotherapy since the early 1990s. The first edition of *Mindfulness and Psychotherapy* (Germer, Siegel, & Fulton, 2005) arose out of this
ongoing dialogue. During a conversation about revising that volume,
we realized that, at the time, there was no practical guide showing psychotherapists how to bring mindfulness into their clinical practice. To
respond to that need, we offer this book, a hands-on guide to selecting,
adapting, and incorporating mindfulness practices into psychotherapy.

During the past decade, there has been an explosion of interest in
mindfulness meditation among mental health professionals. Not only
has mindfulness found a place in mainstream psychotherapy, it is now the
fastest-developing area in clinical practice. Many clinicians have come
to view mindfulness as a curative mechanism that transcends diagnosis,

addresses underlying causes of suffering, and is an active ingredient in most effective psychotherapies. The clinical value of mindfulness techniques has been demonstrated for many psychological difficulties, including depression, anxiety, chronic pain, substance abuse, insomnia, and obsessive–compulsive disorder. Interventions have proven effective with a wide range of patients, from individuals with chronic mental illness to children, adolescents, couples, and families.

Mindfulness practice can also aid us as clinicians. It can contribute to our own emotional well-being, helping us develop beneficial therapeutic qualities such as acceptance, attention, equanimity, and attunement that enrich and enliven our work and help us avoid burnout. And once we develop these qualities in ourselves, we can safely and thoughtfully introduce our patients to the clinical benefits of mindfulness. This is true regardless of our therapeutic persuasion— be it psychodynamic, cognitive-behavioral, acceptance-based, relational, systemic, existential, humanistic, or any other. As interest in this approach grows, patients are seeking therapists of all stripes who practice mindfulness themselves and have a mindfulness-informed approach to mental health.

Many clinicians want to incorporate these skills into psychotherapy, but aren't sure how to begin. This book is a good place to start. Historically, mindfulness practices have been presented as one-size-fits-all remedies. However, as the field matures, we're becoming more sophisticated and nuanced in understanding how these practices affect different individuals with different problems at different stages in their development. Through accumulating wisdom from mindfulness training programs, combined with clinical and neurobiological research findings, we are learning how to tailor practices to fit the patient. Therefore, rather than presenting a recipe or a manualized treatment program, we offer guidelines that will help you employ mindfulness practices based on your patients' unique needs as well as on your own therapeutic style and orientation. Toward this end, we present a wide variety of practices that can be further adapted to address particular situations in treatment. As in mindfulness practice itself, our emphasis is on flexibility, "being in the moment," and responding skillfully to whatever arises.

If you don't meditate, this book can help you get started. If you do, it can help you expand and sustain your practice. Building on the foundation of our own personal practice, we outline ways to become a more mindful therapist and cultivate mindfulness in the therapeutic relationship. We then introduce practices to develop the core mind-fulness skills of concentration (focused attention), mindfulness per se (open monitoring), loving-kindness, compassion, and equanimity, and bring these practices to life with varied clinical illustrations. We also suggest ways to modify them for individual patients and to work with the obstacles that often arise. Because it is easy to feel overwhelmed by the large number of mindfulness practices available, we provide guide-lines for how to sequence and combine various practices for optimal benefit.

Sometimes, mindfulness practice draws therapists and patients alike beyond the boundaries of traditional psychotherapy into the realm of personal or spiritual transformation, so we offer suggestions for con-sidering these transitions as well. We also include an appendix with practices and sequences that we have found useful in treating particular disorders and specific clinical populations, as well as resources to delve further into mindfulness practice and its clinical applications.

Because our emphasis is on real-world clinical practice, and because our intention is to make this book as accessible as possible, we have minimized references to research and other academic writings. Those who are interested in the scientific underpinnings of mindful-ness practice can learn more about them in our companion volume, *Mindfulness and Psychotherapy, Second Edition* (Germer, Siegel, & Fulton, 2013). Also, following the convention in that book, we have decided to use the word "patient" instead of "client" throughout this book. Since "patient" means "one who bears suffering" and "doctor" means "teacher," we as psychotherapists can think of ourselves as "doctoring patients," or "teaching people who bear suffering." For mindfulness is, above all else, a teaching meant to alleviate suffering.

Written for clinicians and by clinicians, this book is designed to empower you to incorporate mindfulness into both your professional practice and your personal life. We hope it will be a helpful companion on the journey.

Acknowledgments

The meditation practices in this book have been the fruit of decades of practice and study with many teachers. For their wisdom, compassion, and inspiration, we offer profound thanks to all from whom we've had the privilege of learning, in particular, His Holiness the Dalai Lama, Jack Kornfield, Sharon Salzberg, Joseph Goldstein, Trudy Goodman, Chogyam Trungpa, Pema Chodron, Shunryu Suzuki, Ram Das, Thich Nhat Hahn, Pir Vilayat Khan, Kalu Rinpoche, Sylvia Boorstein, Tara Brach, Narayan Helen Liebenson, Michael Grady, Larry Rosenberg, Michele McDonald, Rodney Smith, Surya Das, and Lama Willa Miller.

We also are grateful for the guidance of many clinical supervisors and professors who have helped us understand the art and science of psychotherapy and the complexities of the human psyche, including our professors during graduate training, as well as colleagues and teachers at Cambridge Health Alliance, Cambridge Youth Guidance Center, South Shore Counseling Center, Harvard University Health Services, Mount Auburn Hospital, and the Schiff Adult Day Treatment Center. In particular, we'd like to thank Robert Bosnak, Dan Brown, Harvey Cox, Thomas Dallamora, Rebecca Drill, Charles Ducey, Diana Eck, Janina Fisher, Howard Gardner, William Geoghegan, Carol Gilligan, George Goethals, Morrie Goodman, Judith Lewis Herman, Rita Hurwitz,

Alfred Margulies, Stan Messer, Linda Miller, Stan Moldawsky, Richard Niebuhr, Barbara Pizer, Nancy Riemer, Richard Schwartz, Bennett Simon, Gerry Stechler, and Merry White.

We'd also like to thank some of the pioneers who have advanced our understanding of mindfulness practices and how they can help with both everyday problems and more serious disorders, including Richard Davidson, Jack Engler, Mark Epstein, Daniel Goleman, Steven Hayes, Jon Kabat-Zinn, Marsha Linehan, Barry Magid, Alan Marlatt, Susan Orsillo, Liz Roemer, Jeffrey Rubin, Zindel Segal, and Daniel Siegel.

Our longtime friends and colleagues at the Institute for Meditation and Psychotherapy (IMP) greatly contributed to our understanding of the interface between these fields. In fact, the idea for this book arose during an IMP board meeting. We thank Doriana Chialant, Paul Fulton, Trudy Goodman, Sara Lazar, Bill Morgan, Stephanie Morgan, Susan Morgan, Andrew Olendzki, Mark Sorensen, Charles Styron, Janet Surrey, and Christopher Willard. We owe special thanks to Christopher Germer, who encouraged us to develop our idea and present it to The Guilford Press, and to Kristy Arbon, who provided invaluable administrative help with the manuscript. We remain grateful to our late friend and colleague Phil Aranow, who worked tirelessly to establish IMP and who encouraged us to get our ideas in print.

We are indebted to Senior Editor Jim Nageotte for his vision, intelligence, and support of this book and so many other clinical books on mindfulness; to Senior Assistant Editor Jane Keislar for her steadfast encouragement; to Senior Production Editor Louise Farkas for help with editorial and production details; and to the many others at Guilford who have contributed to this project. We are particularly grateful to Art Director Paul Gordon for his handsome and evocative cover design and his skill and graciousness in incorporating our input.

Harvard Medical School, Cambridge Health Alliance, has provided a venue where these practices have been taught since 1994. We are grateful to the many students who have given feedback and helped us refine these practices in the laboratory of the clinical hour. We also thank Adam Elias, Deb Hulihan, Liz Gaufberg, and Catherine Schuman for supporting and fostering this work. Colleagues elsewhere have also provided important teaching venues in which to develop our ideas, including Ruth Buczynski, Richard Fields, Rob Guerette, Chip Hartranft, Jack Hirose, Maddy Klyne, Gerry Piaget, Judy Reiner Platt, and Rich Simon.

Our most powerful teachers, however, have been our patients, who have opened their hearts and trusted us with their deepest sorrows. They are the guiding force behind this book. Although their stories are front and center in this guide, their identities have been disguised to protect confidentiality.

Finally, we are indebted to our friends and family who have offered support. While there isn't room to acknowledge them all, we would like to thank the members of the Wednesday meditation group, Matt Czaplinski, Dan Foley, Suzanne Hoffman, Tom Putnam, Ed Yeats, Janet Yassen, and Judi Zoldan, for nearly 20 years of meditation, study, and conversation. Jerome Bass, Elissa Ely, Bo Forbes, Caroline Jones, Barbara Kleeman, Carin Roberge, Sally Anne Schreiber, Niti Seth, Janna Malamud Smith, and Sherry Turkle have provided wise counsel. And, of course, none of this would have been possible without the love and encouragement of our parents, Marianne and Peter Pedulla, Rita and Robert Pollak, and Claire and Sol Siegel; our children, Nathaniel Weisenberg, Hillary Pollak, and Julia and Alexandra Siegel; and other family members, including Faye Levey (who introduced one of us, Susan Pollak, to meditation in elementary school), Maryellen McDonnell, Paul Pedulla, Pete Pedulla, and Rick and Anita Pollak.

We owe the greatest debt to our partners, Christine Aquilino, Gina Arons, and Adam Weisenberg, who have read and commented on rough drafts, provided food and comfort, and tolerated our distracted minds and our more than occasional lack of presence during months of writing.

May many beings benefit from this book.

Contents

Chapter 1. Bringing Mindfulness into Psychotherapy   1

What Exactly Is Mindfulness?   2
The Roles of Mindfulness   2
Not One Size Fits All   4
Meditation Practices as Counterproductive Defenses   20
It's Complicated, but Worth It   26

Chapter 2. Becoming a Mindful Therapist   27

Do Therapists Benefit from Mindfulness Training?   28
Getting Started: The Basics   30
Taking the Next Step   31
Bringing Mindfulness into the Consulting Room   35
What to Do When You're Feeling Discouraged   43
Moving Beyond Us   44

Chapter 3. Cultivating Mindfulness   45
in the Therapeutic Relationship

Deepening Therapeutic Presence   46
Getting Out of the Way   53
Not Knowing   55
Relational Mindfulness   58
Transitioning to Mindfulness-Based Treatment   62

Chapter 4. Concentration Practice: Focusing the Mind   65
            Paying Attention to Posture   67
            Making Concentration Practice Accessible to Patients   67
            What Does Concentration Look and Feel Like?   79

Chapter 5. Open Monitoring: Expanding the Mind   82
            Developing Awareness of the Body   84
            Mindfulness of Emotions   92
            Putting It All Together   97
            It's OK to Lose It   99

Chapter 6. Loving-Kindness and Compassion Practice: 100
            Engaging the Heart
            Bringing Compassion to the Body   105
            Bringing Compassion to Eating   107
            Taking Compassion from the Meditation
               Cushion into the World   110
            Working with Extreme Suffering   111
            When Life Feels Unbearable   116
            The Inner Darth Vader   119

Chapter 7. Equanimity Practice: Finding Balance   120
            You Can't Stop the Waves   124
            Finding a Still Place   127
            Turning toward the Pain   129
            Rethinking Forgiveness   131
            When Only Industrial Strength Will Do   134
            The Most Wondrous Thing   136

Chapter 8. Making Mindfulness Accessible   139
            How to Start   140
            "There's a Tornado in Me"   148
            Nothing Weird   151

Chapter 9. The Art of Sequencing   156
            Working with Things as They Are   158
            Putting It All Together   160

Chapter 10. Beyond Symptom Relief: Deepening Mindfulness   175

Are We Therapists or Meditation Teachers?   177
Deepening Our Own Meditation Practice   177
Deepening Our Patients' Meditation Practice   183

Appendix.   Selecting Practices   195

Practices for Particular Disorders   196
Practices for Particular Populations   200
Practices for the Clinician   202
Additional Practices   202

Resources   213

Books about Mindfulness Meditation   213
Recordings   215
Meditation Centers   216
Mindfulness Training in Clinical Settings   223

References   225

Index   235

CHAPTER ONE

Bringing Mindfulness
into Psychotherapy

The faculty of voluntarily bringing back a wandering
attention, over and over again, is the very root of judgment,
character, and will.
                        —WILLIAM JAMES (1890/2007, p. 424)

Mindfulness is a deceptively simple way of relating to experience that has been practiced for over 2,500 years to alleviate human
suffering. In recent years, clinicians are discovering that mindfulness
holds great promise for both their own personal development and as a
way to enhance therapeutic relationships. It is also the central ingredient in an ever-expanding range of empirically supported treatments,
and it is proving to be a remarkably powerful technique to augment
virtually every form of psychotherapy. Mindfulness is not, however, a
one-size-fits-all remedy. Practices need to be tailored to fit the needs
of particular individuals and situations. This chapter explores the varied
roles that mindfulness can play in psychotherapy and the choices we
clinicians face in fitting practices to our own and our patients' changing needs.

1

WHAT EXACTLY IS MINDFULNESS?

As used by Western psychotherapists, the term *mindfulness* is often understood to be a translation of the Pali term *sati* (Pali is the language in which the teachings of the historical Buddha were first recorded). *Sati* connotes *awareness, attention,* and *remembering.* Awareness and attention here are similar to how we use them in English—to be aware and to pay attention. *Remembering* is different, however. Rather than remembering what we had for breakfast or recalling childhood trauma, it refers to continuously remembering to be aware and pay attention.

As we use it in psychotherapy, mindfulness also includes another essential dimension. The Buddhist scholar John Dunne (2007) points out that a Special Forces sniper poised on top of a building aiming a high-powered rifle at an enemy would be aware and attentive, and each time his mind wandered, he'd remember to return his attention to the task at hand. But this kind of focus is probably not optimal for developing therapeutic presence or working effectively with emotional distress. What's missing for the sniper is acceptance or nonjudgment—adding an attitude of warmth, friendliness, and compassion. (We might think of this as adding in the Rogers—Carl and Mister.) So putting these elements together, we can think of mindfulness as *"awareness* of *present experience* with *acceptance"* (Germer, 2013, p. 7) or "the awareness that emerges through paying attention on purpose, and nonjudgmentally, to the unfolding of experience moment to moment" (Kabat-Zinn, 2003, p. 145). Of particular importance for psychotherapy is the attitude of acceptance: "active nonjudgmental embracing of experience in the here and now" (Hayes, 2004, p. 21).

THE ROLES OF MINDFULNESS

Mindfulness can play a variety of roles in psychotherapy. We can conceptualize these roles along a continuum, from implicit to explicit (Germer, 2013; Figure 1.1). At the most implicit end of the continuum is the practicing therapist. When we take up regular mindfulness practice, we naturally begin to relate differently to our patients. As the mind's capacity for attention increases, it becomes easier to truly show up in the therapy room and to focus the mind and notice the moment-to-moment unfolding of both our patients' and our own thoughts

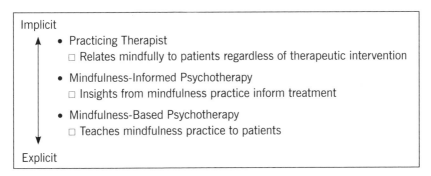

FIGURE 1.1. The roles of mindfulness.

and feelings. We also develop greater affect tolerance—an enhanced capacity to *be with* painful feelings. By being with and accepting both pleasurable and painful experiences during mindfulness practice, we increase our ability to sit with our patients' difficulties, as well as our emotional responses to these difficulties (Fulton, 2013). And as we explore in Chapter 3, the therapist's capacity to open to emotional distress is key to effective therapeutic relationships.

Next along the continuum is what we and our colleagues call *mindfulness-informed* psychotherapy. As our own mindfulness practice deepens, we begin to gain firsthand insight into how our minds create suffering. We notice, for example, that any experience or mental content that we resist tends to persist. We see how attempts at self-aggrandizement, clinging to pleasure, and trying to avoid pain all create distress. We see how much of our energies are spent seeking momentary distraction from discomfort. These and related observations begin to influence our models of psychopathology and treatment, as we notice that our patients' minds create suffering in similar ways. Our treatments become increasingly oriented toward helping our patients open to and accept a wider range of experience.

At the most explicit end of the continuum is what we and our colleagues call *mindfulness-based* psychotherapy. Here we suggest to some of our patients, when clinically appropriate, that they try mindfulness practices themselves. Based initially on our own practice experience, we introduce techniques that are suited to each patient's personality structure, level of distress, degree of support, and cultural orientation. Often these techniques are first practiced together in the office and then suggested as homework between sessions.

NOT ONE SIZE FITS ALL

We had the privilege some years ago of having His Holiness the Dalai Lama join us at Harvard Medical School for a psychotherapy conference. At one point our colleague, Chris Germer, asked His Holiness to lead us all in a brief meditation. In his inimitable style, the Dalai Lama (2009) reacted as though the request was funny: "I think some of you may want just one single meditation. And a simple one. And 100 percent sort of positive. That, I think, impossible." He went on to suggest that there are countless states of mind that lead to suffering and, consequently, countless meditation practices that are needed to work skillfully with them. What a given person needs at a given time is a complicated matter. He concluded, "Some other sort of companies, they always advertise some simple thing, or something effective, something very cheap. My advertising is just opposite. How difficult, and complicated!"

Whether we are choosing practices for ourselves or our patients, deciding which practice will be most useful at a given moment for a particular individual is indeed a complex matter. Clinicians are just beginning to map this territory, without much data to guide us. Practices that support the development of mindfulness can be found in many different cultures, and most of these practices have evolved extensively over time. Furthermore, individual clinicians will naturally experiment with mixing and modifying practices for the needs of particular patients. An extraordinarily wide variety of practices are therefore available to us.

While there are countless ways to categorize and describe these practices, based on our clinical experience we've identified seven considerations clinicians might keep in mind when choosing among them:

1. Which skills to emphasize—concentration, open monitoring (mindfulness per se), or acceptance?
2. Informal, formal, or retreat practice?
3. Which objects of attention—coarse or subtle?
4. Religious or secular practices?
5. Turning toward safety or sharp points?
6. Narrative or experiential focus?
7. Focus on relative or absolute truth?

Let's examine these considerations, and see how we might use them to develop guidelines for when to choose which form of practice.

Which Skills to Emphasize?

Developing mindfulness involves at least three major skills: *focused attention* (or concentration), *open monitoring* (or mindfulness per se), and *compassionate acceptance* (Lutz, Slagter, Dunne, & Davidson, 2008; Germer, 2013). (These terms can be confusing because in Buddhist traditions, open monitoring is usually called "mindfulness," whereas in the West we typically use the word *mindfulness* as an umbrella term covering a variety of interrelated practices.) Focused attention, in which we choose an object of awareness and follow it closely, is usually a good place for most people to start. These practices focus and stabilize the mind, forming a foundation for developing other skills. While the primary object of awareness can be virtually anything, including sensations of the breath, feet touching the ground, sounds, or a visual stimulus, overall instructions are usually similar. We bring our attention to the object, attempting to cultivate an attitude of interest or curiosity in moment-to-moment sensations. As thoughts enter the mind—which they invariably will—we allow them to arise and pass. When our minds get hijacked by a chain of narrative thought, or wander to other sensations, we gently redirect our focus back to the primary object of attention. (Note that "concentration" as described here is different from "concentrating" on a conceptual or creative task. It's not about the focused application of analytical or artistic skill, or thinking through a problem, but rather careful, receptive attention to moment-to-moment experiences arising in consciousness.) Chapter 4 presents detailed instructions for these practices.

Without a certain degree of concentration, it becomes difficult to see the workings of the mind clearly. We tend instead to spend our days lost in thought. When involved in our verbal narratives, we usually both believe in their content and lose metacognitive awareness of what the mind is doing in each moment. Without concentration, it is also difficult to exercise choice in our behavior—we tend to act compulsively on impulses, not noticing that we have an opportunity to pause and consider our responses before pursuing pleasure or recoiling from pain. Finally, without concentration, it is also quite difficult to practice the other two skills necessary for developing mindfulness: open monitoring and compassionate acceptance.

Once a certain degree of focused attention or concentration has developed, and the mind can stay with an object for a little while and realize when it has wandered off, it becomes possible to practice open monitoring. Here, instead of returning repeatedly to one object of awareness—such as the sensations of breathing or of the feet touching the ground—we turn our focus to whatever predominates in consciousness at the moment. Attention might shift from the breath to a sound, to a body ache, to the feeling of air on the face, or to sensations of sadness in the eyes and throat. Rather than thinking about or analyzing these sensations, we allow the mind to *be with* them, bringing an attitude of interest, curiosity, and acceptance to the experience. Until a person has spent some time developing concentration and knows what it is like to remain with a single object of attention for a period of time, it can be difficult to get a feel for open monitoring. The attitude is sometimes described as like sitting next to a still forest pool to which all sorts of creatures come to drink before they move on. Which creatures will arrive, and when they will leave, is quite beyond our control. We therefore try to welcome them all. Detailed instructions for these practices are presented in Chapter 5.

One way to understand the relationship between focused attention and open monitoring is by thinking about photography before cameras were automated. In those days, to get a clear picture, you first had to know how to focus the camera lens. Without this skill, a photographer was limited to abstract, impressionistic, blurry images. Learning to concentrate is like focusing the mind's lens—it allows us to see clearly whatever we turn our attention to. Once this skill is developed, we can use it to examine whatever might be happening at the moment.

Open monitoring can be useful for seeing how the mind creates suffering as it resists various sensory experiences as well as emerging thoughts or images. It is also helpful for reintegrating previously split-off or disavowed contents. These contents can include thoughts, feelings, and impulses that aren't sanctioned by our families or wider community, or memories of traumatic events that were too painful to experience fully when they occurred. Open monitoring helps us notice these contents as they arise in the mind, and as we practice greeting them with acceptance, they can become familiar and no longer feel like foreign intrusions. Just as in psychoanalysis, where if one lies on the couch and freely says whatever comes to mind, sooner or later a lot of material that we've tried to avoid will emerge—so too in mindfulness practice such contents will tend to return to awareness. What emerges can range from minor traumatic memories, such as moments of rejection or failure, to major ones, such as experiences of physical or sexual abuse. Aggressive, avaricious, and sexual impulses that we think of as immoral will often also arise. As we'll discuss shortly, such encounters can be useful or damaging, depending on a person's readiness to accept and integrate these contents.

Yet another potential benefit of practicing open monitoring is enhancing our appreciation for the richness of the moment. When we practice attending to sensory experience in meditation, during the rest of our day we tend to taste, touch, see, feel, and smell things more vividly, increasing our capacity to savor experience and deeply enriching our day-to-day life.

Concentration and mindfulness work well together to cultivate attention and awareness. But in the course of these practices, people often become overwhelmed by the intensity of what arises or find themselves trapped in self-critical patter. In these moments, more acceptance is needed. Loving-kindness, self-compassion, and equanimity techniques can be useful at these times for holding and soothing, fortifying us to be able to bear whatever we might experience.

Acceptance practices take many forms. A common type involves imagining a loving and compassionate person or animal, directing love and care toward him or her, and then, once feeling this emotion, directing it as well toward oneself, loved ones, and larger communities. The feeling is often reinforced with phrases such as *May you be happy, May you be peaceful, May you be free from suffering*. Similar practices, with parallels to prayer, can be drawn from a variety of cultural traditions. They all help people to feel loved, held, and accepting of themselves and others. Other acceptance practices include compassion techniques designed to help us feel held during times of emotional pain and equanimity practices that enhance our capacity to bear or hold challenging experiences, cultivating stability amid storms of changing emotion. Detailed instructions for these various acceptance practices are presented in Chapters 6 and 7.

Finding an optimal balance among concentration, mindfulness, and acceptance practices at any given moment is an art. When the mind is particularly frisky and unfocused or tending to get lost in streams of thought, more concentration practice is often helpful. When it is flooded by difficult memories or emotions, or full of self-critical contents, loving-kindness, self-compassion, or equanimity practices often help. When the mind is more stable and accepting, open monitoring can move us toward greater insight and integration by helping us become conscious and accepting of a wide variety of thoughts, feelings, and memories that might otherwise escape our awareness (R. D. Siegel, 2010). Whether in our personal meditation practice or in designing practices for patients, it is useful to be familiar with and willing to try these different sorts of practice. Sometimes we might spend an entire period of meditation with one type, while at other times we might move among them during the course of a single meditation session, adjusting as our state of mind shifts.

It can also be helpful to think of and use the three core skills as different ways to strengthen the three components of mindfulness (*awareness* of *present-moment experience* with *acceptance*). Concentration practice helps us stay connected to the present moment, open monitoring enables us to broaden and deepen our awareness of what's actually happening in that moment, and loving-kindness and compassion practices allow us to meet all that arises in consciousness with acceptance.

Informal, Formal, or Retreat Practice?

Cultivating mindfulness is a bit like developing physical fitness. Without radically changing our lifestyle, we could take the stairs instead of the elevator, or ride our bike instead of driving, and develop some physical fitness. To become more fit, however, we'd need to take time out of our daily routine and go to the gym, go jogging, or play a sport. If we really want to jump-start our fitness program, we might even go away for several days on a bike or backpacking trip or take a vacation at an exercise spa. Analogous options are available for developing mindfulness: informal, formal, and retreat practice.

Without taking extra time out of our day, we can adopt *informal* mindfulness practices such as mindfully walking, showering, eating, or driving. These only require a shift in intention. For example, in mindful walking, instead of having our attention focused on what happened in yesterday's meeting, or on planning dinner, we notice the moment-to-moment sensations of our feet touching the ground and moving forward through space. In mindful showering, we savor the intense sensual experience of thousands of drops of water—at just the right temperature—caressing our naked bodies. We take in the vivid sensations of washing, soaping, and rinsing ourselves, rather than reviewing our to-do list and reaching the end of our shower with no idea whether we have just washed our hair, "Or was that yesterday?" In mindful eating we try to taste our food, and in mindful driving we notice the appearance of the road, other cars, trees, houses, and so forth. In all of these activities, when thoughts enter the mind, we allow them to come and go, returning attention to the sensations of this moment's activity. Anyone can develop some mindfulness through these sorts of informal practices since they require no extra time and are rarely destabilizing.

But if we want to deepen our mindfulness practice, we need the equivalent of the gym. This is time set aside for *formal* meditation. We choose a quiet place where we're unlikely to be disturbed to do some combination of focused attention, open monitoring, and acceptance practices. These practice sessions can range from brief periods of 10–20 minutes to more intensive ones of 30–45 minutes. Studies demonstrating changes in brain function and structure from mindfulness practice typically investigate the effects of such formal meditation practice, and most mindfulness-based clinical protocols include it (Lazar, 2013).

Many patients have difficulty engaging in formal practice. As we mentioned earlier, meditation can open the doors to all sorts of unwanted mental contents that can be difficult to bear. Longer periods of silent practice, particularly if focused on the breath, can become overwhelming. People also may feel they have no time—their lives are already too full with other commitments. Still others may see meditation as an alien practice that runs counter to their religious or cultural beliefs. As we'll see, however, most of these obstacles can be overcome by finding the right combination and intensity of practices and presenting them in a culturally sensitive, collaborative manner.

To really jump-start a meditation practice, there's nothing like an intensive silent retreat: spending a day or more alternating among sitting, walking, eating, and other meditation practices. We refrain from eye contact with others, speaking, reading, writing, texting, and checking e-mail. Retreats tend to shift our level of mindfulness significantly, and most participants find them to be radically transformational.

In fact, it is difficult to grasp the potential of mindfulness practice fully without experiencing a silent retreat. It is hard to develop sufficient concentration during the course of daily practice to observe the workings of the mind clearly. During everyday life we need to spend a lot of time thinking and planning to accomplish our goals. As a result, we dwell mostly in the thought stream, our continuous verbal narrative about our experience.

During an intensive silent retreat, however, there are few decisions needed and few goals, other than cultivating mindfulness, to pursue. As a result the mind tends to quiet down, and spaces often open up between thoughts. We get to see how the mind creates its understanding of reality out of the building blocks of sensation, perception, feelings, and intentions. We see over and over how trying to hold on to pleasurable experiences and push away painful ones causes suffering. And we may even get a glimpse into the insubstantiality of our sense of self—how it is constructed each moment out of an endlessly changing flux of experience. These insights have enormous potential to change our understanding of psychological distress, whether as therapists or as patients.

But they also pose significant dangers. A few decades ago, Western meditation teachers rarely screened for psychological stability before allowing people to enroll in intensive retreats and quite a few meditators suffered psychotic breaks. There were many cases in which we and our colleagues were enlisted by meditation teachers or participants to provide consultation or treatment. For individuals with a fragile or rigid sense of self, significant unresolved or unintegrated trauma, or who might be suffering from psychosis, silent retreats are usually contraindicated. While some meditation centers have since developed guidelines for whom to allow to attend intensive retreats, many participants still become overwhelmed when their habitual defenses are challenged. Evaluating who among our patients is most suited for intensive practice requires both considerable personal retreat experience and a good understanding of our patients' strengths and vulnerabilities. This understanding can best be gathered through a treatment relationship in which we observe the extent to which our patient can open to and accept the varied contents of his or her mind, his or her affect tolerance, and how readily he or she can let go of cognitive frameworks through which to understand experiences. It is also important to consider patients' biopsychosocial resources, including the strength of the therapeutic alliance, availability of support from family and friends, degree of safety in daily life, quality of early attachment relationships, and genetic predisposition toward psychiatric disorders. The more risk factors that are present, the more cautious we should be about recommending retreat practice. Chapter 10 presents more details about screening for and participating in retreat practice.

Which Objects of Attention?

In concentration practice, we can choose to focus on subtle objects of attention, such as the sensation of the breath entering and leaving the nostrils, or more vivid, coarse objects, such as the sensations of the soles of the feet touching the ground when walking (see Figure 1.2).

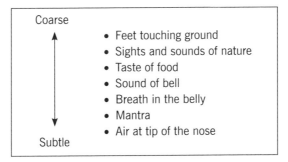

Coarse
- Feet touching ground
- Sights and sounds of nature
- Taste of food
- Sound of bell
- Breath in the belly
- Mantra
- Air at tip of the nose
Subtle

FIGURE 1.2. Objects of attention.

When the mind is friskier and more distracted, coarser objects are easier to follow. So why don't we always choose coarse objects of attention for formal meditation practice? Why do so few of us go to heavy metal concerts to meditate? After all, it's easy to attend to the principal objects of attention there, the sound and light. In fact, it's likely that many fans attend such concerts precisely because they enjoy the experience of absorption—of setting aside their usual thoughts and feelings and being engrossed in the loud music and compelling visuals. The problem is, we don't seem to develop refined attention with such vivid objects; we can attend to the stimuli, but it is not so easy also to notice what's happening in the mind and to attain insight. We don't readily see the mind's tendency to hold on to some contents while pushing away others, observe subtle feelings, or notice how the mind reacts to loss and gain.

So in clinical practice, as well as in our personal meditation, we need to choose when to select more subtle objects and when to select coarser ones. Many meditators find that coarser objects are useful when the mind has difficulty staying with a chosen object of awareness, when thoughts repeatedly pull attention away. They are also helpful when our arousal state is high, as in moments of increased anxiety or excitement. While different individuals may experience one or another object as more or less vivid, for most people, noticing the sensations of the feet in walking meditation, or the sights and sounds of nature, the taste of food, or the sound of a bell will help stabilize the mind when the mind is active or agitated. When the mind is more settled, less aroused, and less drawn toward thought, more subtle objects of attention such as the sensation of the breath entering and leaving the nostrils, the rising and falling of the belly, or a mantra (silently repeated phrases) may allow for more refined attention.

Religious or Secular Practices?

Clinicians in many parts of the United States regularly ask, "How can I introduce my religiously conservative clients to these practices? They'll reject anything that comes from Buddhism or is called 'meditation.'" Some years ago, the Dalai Lama (2007) was talking to researchers studying depression. He suggested that if they discovered that particular Buddhist practices can help depressed people, the researchers shouldn't emphasize that they come from Buddhism. He went on to say that the whole purpose of his tradition is to alleviate suffering, and if people think of these practices as Buddhist, such thinking will just get in the way.

All effective psychotherapy requires sensitivity to patients' cultural background. This becomes particularly true when introducing practices that have been adapted from traditions that are alien to our patients' beliefs. With secular, scientifically minded individuals, the path is relatively straightforward. We now have an impressive body of neurobiological and clinical outcomes research to point to that describe these mindfulness practices in Western scientific terms. And for secular patients who might be disturbed by the Buddhist roots of some of these practices, we can follow the lead of John Teasdale, Zindel Segal, and Mark Williams (1995), when they first published papers about using mindfulness practice as part of depression treatment, and simply call it *attentional control training,* which it is.

For more religiously inclined patients, deciding how to present these practices is more complicated. We need first to assess their openness to other traditions. Sometimes a practice adapted from another religious tradition is more appealing than one coming from a secular, scientific source. In this case presenting some of these practices as coming from a Buddhist tradition may not be a problem.

Alternatively, we can look for mindfulness practices related to our patient's particular religious background. For example, we can offer *centering prayer* techniques from medieval Catholic monastic traditions (Pennington, 1980), as well as modern adaptations of Kabalistic Jewish (Michaelson, 2006) and Sufi Muslim (Helminski, 1992) practices (see the Resources).

Of course, like secular individuals, some religious patients will do best with a nonreligious presentation of these practices. If we avoid words with religious associations such as *meditation* and present these practices as the tools they are for cognitive development, mental training, or harnessing neuroplasticity, our patients can accept mindfulness practices as readily as other medical interventions or educational offerings. We've heard accounts, for example, of mindfulness practices being successfully introduced to patients in evangelical religious communities as attention training—a way to focus more clearly at church, work, and school.

Although these practices can be framed in many different ways, there may be a point when a mindfulness-oriented approach to treatment is difficult to reconcile with a particular faith tradition. This occurs most frequently when the religious tradition teaches that certain contents of mind are to be eliminated because they are "sinful." Here it can be helpful to enlist the assistance of clergy who emphasize the more accepting or loving elements in their tradition, or to explore with our patient the pros and cons of a prohibitionary approach to potentially problematic thoughts, feelings, and impulses.

Turning toward Safety or Sharp Points?

Most clinicians are sensitive to the challenge of titrating interventions—not pushing patients too quickly into uncomfortable, potentially destabilizing waters. We have general agreement, born from studying trauma, that people need to establish safety before either uncovering repressed memories or moving toward disavowed thoughts and feelings (e.g., Herman, 1992; van der Kolk, McFarlane, & Weisaeth, 1996).

As mentioned earlier, our interpersonal milieu often discourages us from acknowledging certain mental contents. A boy might grow up fearing that his longings for love and affection or feelings of vulnerability make him a "sissy," whereas a girl might be concerned that her assertiveness makes her a "tomboy." Many people are raised to feel that all sorts of sexual, acquisitive, or aggressive feelings are immoral. On top of this, most of us have had overwhelming experiences in which our hearts were broken or we were shamed, threatened, or physically injured. Such events may have been only partially experienced at the time because they were too painful to bear, and memories of them may now be only partly accessible. Exploring such material in therapy needs to be done thoughtfully so as not to overwhelm or retraumatize our patients.

It turns out that some meditation practices generally enhance safety and allow difficult contents to be kept at bay, while others move people toward thoughts, feelings, and memories that may have been disavowed—what is called in Tibetan Buddhist tradition *moving toward the sharp points*. While we don't yet have experimental data indicating which practices typically yield which effects, we can look to existing therapy traditions for some guidance.

Generally, it seems that meditation practices that bring our attention to the chest, belly, and throat (such as attending to the sensations of the breath) move us toward the sharp points, while those that focus on objects farther away (such as the soles of the feet, sounds, the taste of food, or the natural environment) tend to be more stabilizing. This principle is related to the observation from Eugene Gendlin's (1978) focusing method and other body-oriented psychotherapies, that paying attention to body sensations in the chest, belly, and throat connects us readily with salient memories and affects, turning our attention toward the sharp points. We've seen repeatedly in both personal and clinical experience how simply closing one's eyes and noticing sensations in the central core of the body can provide access to feelings that might otherwise be outside of awareness.

So if a patient is having difficulty tolerating the intensity of his or her affect or is feeling overwhelmed by intrusive thoughts or images, choosing "external" objects of attention and using them in concentration practice, can provide an experience of grounding or safety without intensifying awareness of challenging "inner" contents. All of these more "external" sensations involve a focus away from the core of the body and can be done as informal (during the course of other activities) or formal (setting time aside for meditation) practices. They include walking, listening, observing the outside environment, and eating meditations, practiced with the eyes open. In essence, we help our patients to realize that whatever may be arising inside, the relatively safe sensations of the outer world can provide a welcome refuge.

In addition to externally focused concentration practices, certain mindfulness-building techniques involving imagery can provide stabilization. Mindfulness involves awareness of present experience with acceptance and these practices are designed specifically to fortify our capacity for acceptance, for allowing painful feelings to come and go. The techniques don't bring attention either to the core of the body or to external sensations, but rather focus on cultivating particular feelings or perspectives. The loving-kindness and self-compassion practices described in detail in Chapter 6 work in this way to help people feel soothed and comforted, particularly when overwhelmed by painful feelings. Similarly, guided imagery techniques, such as the mountain meditation (in which we imagine ourselves as a mountain being relatively steady as seasonal changes occur on and around us—see Chapter 7 for a description), can cultivate equanimity, providing a sense of stability amid changing emotional and environmental circumstances. Zen techniques used in dialectical behavior therapy (DBT; Linehan, 1993a, 1993b), such as coordinating the breath with footsteps, imagining the mind as a vast sky in which contents arise and pass, or adopting a serene half-smile, can also help people to feel safer.

When a patient is in a relatively stable life situation, has a good therapeutic alliance, and is not overwhelmed by affect or difficult memories, it may be time to help him or her move toward the sharp points: to confront troubling memories, explore uncomfortable feelings, or perhaps look at the consequences of problematic behaviors. This means approaching and reintegrating affects, impulses, images, and memories that may have been pushed out of awareness because of their painful nature. While there are many psychotherapeutic techniques useful for this kind of uncovering, certain mindfulness practices can be particularly effective.

As mentioned above, if a meditator spends sufficient time attending to an inner object of awareness, such as the breath, sooner or later a wide range of disavowed mental contents usually will come into awareness. While this reaction can occur during concentration practice, it is even more likely to happen with open monitoring.

Most people find that once they decide to shift their attention toward the sharp points, they are best able to open to and accept the fear, sadness, anger, longing, sexual feelings, and other contents that arise by focusing on how they are experienced, moment to moment, as sensations in the body, typically arising in the torso or throat. When we observe emotions objectively in this way, we notice that they involve the simultaneous arising of bodily sensations along with narrative thoughts and images. So if I'm angry, I might experience the tensing of muscles in my shoulders and chest, an uptick in my respiration and heart rate, and thoughts like, "I can't believe you did that to me after all I've done for you," passing through my mind. By staying with the bodily components of the emotion, rather than the narrative, I'm able to experience it more fully without feeling compelled to take action to "fix" the situation (as I might if I were attending primarily to the narrative content). Most people can tolerate intense affects once they learn to be with them simply as bodily sensations while allowing the accompanying images and narrative thoughts to arise and pass. We can learn to adopt this attitude not only toward emotions but also toward urges for destructive behaviors such as addictions and compulsions (Brewer, 2013; R. D. Siegel, 2010; see also Chapter 7). Figure 1.3 summarizes practices that can be used to establish safety and practices that can be used to move toward the sharp points.

Narrative or Experiential Focus?

Most patients come to treatment wanting to share their stories. They've had good and bad fortune, giving rise to pleasurable and painful thoughts and feelings. Psychotherapy often focuses on this narrative, either to put it in perspective by exploring its origins and subsequent manifestations in the transference and daily life (in psychodynamic treatment); by examining it for irrational, maladaptive distortions (in cognitive-behavioral approaches); or by seeking to understand it in cultural or interpersonal context (in systemic therapies). Focusing on the narrative helps our patients to feel understood and held and can free them from unnecessarily painful mental constructions (Fulton & Siegel, 2013).

Mindfulness practices generally turn attention away from our narratives and toward moment-to-moment experience. Consequently, mindfulness-oriented psychotherapy usually focuses on what is happening here and now, grounded in attention to changing bodily sensations. As just mentioned, learning to pay attention to present bodily sensations can help patients develop greater equanimity and affect tolerance, for emotions are easier to embrace when we experience them in the body, separated from our narrative. Focusing on body sensations can also help to recover traumatic memories or blocked affects, as is done in body-oriented therapies such as somatic experiencing (Levine & Frederick, 1997), sensorimotor therapy (Ogden, Minton, & Pain, 2006), or approaches such as bioenergetics (Lowen, 1958, 1994) that grew out of the work of Wilhelm Reich.

Both approaches are useful. As mindfulness-oriented clinicians, we're regularly challenged to choose between a more traditional narrative focus and a more experiential one. For example, if a young woman is afraid to go to a party because of her social anxiety, practicing staying with the sensations of anxiety in the body, rather than trying to avoid

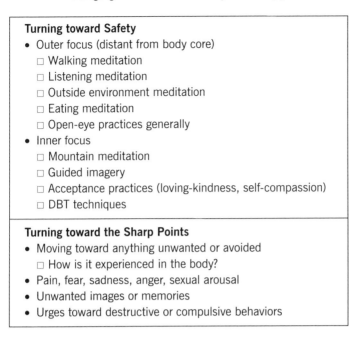

Turning toward Safety
- Outer focus (distant from body core)
  - ☐ Walking meditation
  - ☐ Listening meditation
  - ☐ Outside environment meditation
  - ☐ Eating meditation
  - ☐ Open-eye practices generally
- Inner focus
  - ☐ Mountain meditation
  - ☐ Guided imagery
  - ☐ Acceptance practices (loving-kindness, self-compassion)
  - ☐ DBT techniques

Turning toward the Sharp Points
- Moving toward anything unwanted or avoided
  - ☐ How is it experienced in the body?
- Pain, fear, sadness, anger, sexual arousal
- Unwanted images or memories
- Urges toward destructive or compulsive behaviors

FIGURE 1.3. Techniques for turning toward safety versus the sharp points.

them, can be quite therapeutic. Similarly, if an older man is agitated and shut down in depression, focusing on his underlying sadness and anger as bodily events can begin to reconnect him with his emotional life and traumatic memories that may be contributing to his distress.

Then again, sometimes just staying with moment-to-moment experience is less powerful than exploring the narrative. If a teenage boy is tormented by shame because he acted impulsively, and now fears that his community will shun him, reviewing what happened, examining the conditions that led to his impulsive action, and discussing exactly how he imagines others now see him can provide enormous relief—light and air can go a long way toward resolving shame. A narrative approach may be much more helpful to him than staying with how the experience of shame manifests in his body while he remains mired in self-critical thoughts.

Deciding on the optimal balance between these two approaches is an art. Sometimes we sense that a patient is in touch with feeling experience but is laboring under a particularly irrational, painful narrative—such as a parent who is devastated that his son wasn't accepted at his alma matter. Exploring the story directly, examining what the rejection means to the parent, and how it resonates with other disappointments, may be most useful here. At other times, a person's narrative may not be particularly distorted, or he or she may be locked in patterns of avoidance, so practicing being with moment-to-moment experience may be more freeing. A mother who is afraid to feel her anger at her abusive adolescent daughter, for fear that the anger will further disrupt the relationship, may need to spend some time simply noticing the anger arising in waves in her body. Of course, both approaches might be helpful in any given session—our challenge is to discern when to emphasize one or the other.

While deciding on which approach to emphasize at any given moment will depend on many factors, an overriding consideration might be the extent to which an individual has gravitated toward one or the other mode of dealing with experience. Particularly if a patient seems to be stuck in a pattern of mental suffering, and he or she tends to explore this exclusively with either a narrative or experiential focus, investigating the other approach may help to move the therapeutic process forward.

Relative or Absolute Truth?

Clinicians who delve more deeply into mindfulness practices see a potential that extends far beyond symptom alleviation (see Germer & Siegel, 2012, and Chapter 10 for more details). After all, many of these practices were originally designed for a radical transformation of the mind, a liberation sometimes referred to as enlightenment. This awakening involves looking beyond our usual concepts to see the world as it really is, to be fully aware of what are called in the Buddhist tradition the three characteristics of existence: *anicca*—everything is a constantly changing flux of matter and energy; *dukkha*, often translated as "life is suffering"—the observation that the mind is always dissatisfied, clinging to pleasure and trying to avoid pain; and *anatta*, the realization that if we observe our experience carefully, there's no "I" to be found—no little homunculus inside—just the unfolding moment to moment of sensations and other experiences along with the mind's running narrative commentary about it all (or as the neuroscientist Wolf Singer, 2005, says, the mind is "an orchestra without a conductor").

Directly understanding and embracing these existential realities, which we can think of as absolute truth, brings about enormous free-dom, as we become much less invested in trying to cling to pleasure and avoid pain, enhance our self-esteem, and insist on particular outcomes. Mindfulness-informed therapy has the potential to lead a patient to see these truths. The important clinical questions are how and when.

If a patient enters treatment grieving because his fiancée broke off their engagement shortly before the wedding, pointing out that every-thing changes, so he shouldn't have expected the relationship to last; that we can never hold onto anything; that the mind inevitably creates suffering during good and bad times anyway, so even if he had gotten married he'd have found something else to be distressed about; and that both he and his fiancée are really just changing constellations of mat-ter and energy, with no real existence except as culturally conditioned constructs—this response would probably be experienced as a terrible empathic failure.

Nonetheless, there are moments in treatment when recognizing the futility of our conventional view can be quite useful. Many patients can benefit by seeing how fruitless it is to try to maintain positive self-esteem (we can't all always be above average), how clinging to pleasure and pushing away pain multiplies our misery, and how our experi-ence of life really is all a passing show. In a rather striking example, a patient of ours who had lost her husband some months earlier to cancer and had grieved deeply, shared the following observation: "Sometimes when I'm talking with a friend, I have this realization that it doesn't actually matter that my husband died. While taking in the sight, sound, and feeling of my friend's presence, instead of having the thought 'He's back home,' I have the thought 'He's no longer alive.' All that's actu-ally different in that moment is the thought; the rest of the experience of talking is actually the same." While of course we'd never want to prematurely coax a patient toward this perspective, opening to its pos-sibility can be profoundly liberating.

Psychotherapy almost always needs to begin at the level of what we might call relative reality, which consists of the usual elements of the human story: success and failure, pleasure and pain, longing, hurt, anger, envy, joy, and pride. As therapists, we try to meet our patients where they are at the moment, empathically understanding their emo-tional and cognitive reactions to the ups and downs of life. But once we've established this empathic connection and explored the details of how a patient's particular circumstance might be causing him or her emotional pain, we can consider whether for this patient a broader perspective, a focus on our shared existential predicament and how the mind creates suffering generally, or the realization that all that ever exists is the present moment, might be liberating.

Deciding between relative and absolute levels of understanding is another area in which therapy is more art than science, and we need to draw on the insights revealed in our own mindfulness practice, coupled with clinical experience, for guidance. In general, it makes sense to begin treatment at the level of relative truth and remain there until the patient has been able to explore multiple aspects of whatever experience is difficult, connecting to her or his thoughts and feelings about it. We might consider this exploration to have occurred when the thoughts and feelings that continue to arise feel familiar and are no longer resisted. Once this occurs, if our patient is flexible cognitively and able to entertain multiple viewpoints simultaneously, it could be helpful to explore his or her experiences from a more existential, constructivist vantage point that considers the reality of *anicca*, *dukkha*, and *anatta*.

MEDITATION PRACTICES AS COUNTERPRODUCTIVE DEFENSES

One of the remarkable qualities of the human mind is its creativity in devising psychological defenses. Like the primate who randomly encounters a stick and notices by chance that it's a wonderful tool for picking up tasty ants, our minds learn to use an astonishing range of tricks to avoid discomfort. While some of these are very helpful, in that they allow us to function during difficult circumstances, others get in the way of our growth, development, and optimal functioning. Meditation is no exception. It turns out that virtually all types of mindfulness practice can be used maladaptively as defenses.

Clinging to Concentration

A colleague of ours recalls taking enthusiastically to meditation practice as a young man:

Cliff was shy and awkward, had recently lost his mother, and often felt insecure in social situations. In his commitment to practice, he tried to be mindful throughout the day. So when he was at a party, he would bring his attention to the moment-to-moment sensations of breathing, and whenever his mind wandered off, such as into grieving over his mother, he'd bring it back to his breath. Rather than opening to whatever arose in the mind (open monitoring), or allowing himself to pay attention to the people he was with, whenever painful emotions came up, he focused ever more tightly on his breath. Not surprisingly, he wasn't really able to connect with others or form deep relationships. For him, sticking narrowly to concentration practice had become a counterproductive defense.

Of course, there are times when taking refuge in concentration or another comforting practice (such a loving-kindness meditation) can be quite skillful. When painful emotions or intrusive thoughts or memories are destabilizing, being able to ground our attention in the sensations of the present moment can be a helpful temporary refuge. Our challenge is to sense when such safety is needed and when it stands in the way of growth or optimal functioning.

When a Retreat Becomes an Escape

Other practice choices can also be defensive. For example, while formal meditation and retreats can both be enormously liberating, some people devote their energies to meditation practice to avoid interpersonal commitments or vocational challenges:

Justin had just ended his third marriage due to "irreconcilable differences." Even though he was in his late 50s, his behavior and rage was like that of a young adolescent. He was raised by a mentally ill mother and an alcoholic and physically abusive father. When he was growing up, other children would taunt and pick on him. He was used to being the victim.

Justin couldn't see his role in the demise of his relationships. It was always the fault of the other person. He would end friendships over minor misunderstandings, and his relationships with his mother and sister were also strained, often lapsing into periods without communication. When his therapist tried to make him aware of his contribution to these broken bonds, he saw this observation as aggression and a failure of empathy. He ended treatment, choosing to go to India for an extended meditation retreat. "Therapy" he said, "is not what my heart needs."

Justin apparently hoped that meditation would provide a detour to avoid dealing with developmental and relational difficulties. While the adventure of practicing in India successfully distracted him for a time, painful images of failed relationships began to arise in his mind.

Eventually he realized that he needed to return home to work on connecting with other people.

Trying to discern when intensive practice will be counterproductive is a tricky matter. After all, most clinicians are not monks or nuns—they've chosen to live in a chaotic world of work and love and probably devote only limited time to meditation practice. Yet leaving the hubbub of life as a householder is a choice that has been made by countless renunciates in many spiritual traditions. The founders of most wisdom traditions are said to have taken this path. So when is a person's movement in this direction a considered choice to take his or her psychological and spiritual development to the next level, and when is it a detour to avoid developmental challenge?

As clinicians, we need to be open-minded and aware of our own values to be skillful in understanding such personal decisions. While most of us wouldn't automatically see a turn toward deeper meditation practice as an enactment of unresolved infantile longings to return to a state of oceanic oneness as Freud (1930/2005) did, we might nonetheless be skeptical of others who make major commitments to practice that we have not made ourselves. Or we could err in the other direction—in our enthusiasm for mindfulness practice we might not see how our patient's increased commitment to formal or retreat practice is actually being used to avoid engaging fully in life. Remaining mindful of both possibilities can help us avoid falling prey to either.

Avoiding Uncomfortable Objects of Attention

It is not uncommon to hear, "I really enjoy walking meditation, but I hate sitting practice" (or vice versa). When is it most skillful to choose comfortable objects of attention, and when should we push ourselves (or encourage our patients) toward practices that are more difficult? Some people tend to avoid discomfort and may, as a result, thwart their psychological progress. For example, the patient who prefers walking meditation because he or she doesn't feel anxious or restless while walking may never get to understand and learn to tolerate his or her anxiety or restlessness.

On the other hand, people can adopt an excessively rigid "no pain, no gain" attitude. In this situation, the individual doesn't notice when he or she could use a break from discomfort, when it would be more skillful to choose a practice that feels easier at the moment. Disciplined meditation can be used as a defense against joy, against letting go and being at ease. Listening carefully to our patients' experiences with different techniques, and considering them in the context of their overall personalities, is important for finding a balanced approach to practice.

Downsides of Both Religious and Secular Beliefs

Discussions of how people's religious beliefs, or lack thereof, may support or hinder their psychological development are challenging. There is no objective platform on which to stand. A religiously observant clinician is likely to view these matters differently from a secular one. And yet, this too is an area in which approaches to mindfulness practices can either inhibit or support a patient's growth.

Religious beliefs clearly can provide all sorts of psychological benefits—meaning and purpose, safety, a moral compass, participation in community, and identification with something larger than the individual, to name a few. But they can also bring with them psychological challenges including negative judgments about sexual and aggressive urges, fears of punishment for unacceptable thoughts and feelings, concerns about ostracism, and rigid belief systems.

Strictly secular views often have costs and benefits that are more or less the inverse of those of religious beliefs. Downsides include lack of meaning and purpose, feelings of insecurity and isolation, lack of moral direction, and disconnection from the wider universe. Benefits include greater comfort with our mammalian nature, fewer fears of punishment or concerns about ostracism, and a more flexible or relativistic belief system.

It is possible to take up mindfulness practices in a religious way, which can bring with it the benefits and difficulties that can come with religious devotion. For patients who want to take up mindfulness practice in a religious context, it may be helpful to explore in an open-minded, sensitive manner how a person's religious understanding supports or interferes with his or her psychological development. Does it support him or her in becoming more open and flexible psychologically? Does it help him or her deal with the challenges of existential reality? Similarly, a person who takes up these practices in a rigidly secular way may benefit from seeing how secular beliefs may be helpful or problematic. It can be particularly interesting with more passionately secular individuals to examine how their views may cut them off from noticing their interdependence with the wider world, and how mindfulness practices can be a doorway to the liberating aspects of experiencing this interconnection.

Too Much Safety?

We discussed how taking refuge in focused attention or concentration practice, sticking to comfortable objects of attention, or even devoting excessive time to formal meditation or retreat practice can be used defensively to avoid experiencing challenging life situations or mental contents. On the other hand, turning toward safety can be essential therapeutically, ensuring our practice doesn't traumatize or retraumatize us. Sensing whether more safety or challenge is needed usually requires considerable clinical experience. While it's possible to give rough guidelines as to when cultivating safety is important (unstable living situations; a lot of unintegrated trauma-related thoughts, feelings, and images; a weak therapeutic relationship), it is our experience of working intimately with a wide variety of people that helps us to sense when emotional challenges are too great versus when they're doorways to growth. When students ask us where to get trained as a mindfulness-oriented clinician, we usually suggest that they first become trained broadly as clinicians, working under a trusted supervisor, since developing a sense of when to move someone toward safety or invite him or her into new territory requires intuition informed by experience. We also suggest that they pursue their own mindfulness practice, so that they can see firsthand the effects of various practices while developing the ability to sit with intense emotional experience.

Interestingly, this is an area in which the clinician's own maladaptive defenses can play a big role. If a therapist is afraid of powerful affects, he or she may nudge patients toward safety to avoid his or her own discomfort; if a therapist is insecure about his or her therapeutic talents, and feels a need to show progress, he or she may nudge patients prematurely toward the sharp points.

Lurching Prematurely toward Absolute Truth

Another common danger in taking up mindfulness practice is what is sometimes called the "spiritual bypass." This defensive maneuver occurs most often when people see their practice as part of a spiritual or religious path, leading to wisdom, compassion, connection to God, or enlightenment. Having a purely intellectual understanding of what we've called absolute truth—the changing nature of all phenomena, the way the mind perpetually creates suffering, and the insubstantial nature of our sense of separate self—we deny our human emotions, fooling ourselves into acting as we imagine enlightened or holy people do. So when our friend disappoints us, we immediately turn the other cheek, or notice the suffering behind our friend's behavior, not allowing ourselves to first feel our hurt or anger. The problem with this bypassing of relative reality, like all psychological defenses, is that it drives feelings underground. And when we bury feelings, we seem to bury them alive: they can come back in the form of somatic symptoms, passive–aggressive acts, compulsions, and other maladaptive behavior. Spiritual bypasses are actually moments of mindlessness masquerading as mindfulness—denying our not-so-noble reactions happening in the moment.

Sometimes spiritual bypasses are supported by profound mystical or transcendent experiences that seem to promise a shortcut through life's difficulties. Sooner or later, however, we face the challenges of our ordinary lives—as meditation teacher Jack Kornfield (2000) put it in a book titled *After the Ecstasy, the Laundry.* Unfortunately but understandably, some people would rather skip the laundry altogether:

Sandra had recently returned from a pilgrimage to sacred sites in Asia, where she had a deeply moving "spiritual" experience. She wanted mindfulness-oriented therapy to replicate her epiphany, as well as help with her marriage, her intrusive mother-in-law, and her challenging adolescent son. When her therapist suggested that she look within to begin to observe her mind and her reactions to her family, she became incensed. "I don't want to look within," she said furiously, "I just want them to respect me."

Sandra found that mindfulness practice didn't provide a reliable escape into supernatural or transcendental solutions—despite its potential to powerfully expand our awareness, it doesn't allow us to leapfrog over the challenges of our lives.

As in many of the clinical decisions we've been discussing, here too timing and balance are important considerations. While spiritual bypasses are often countertherapeutic, there is a role for cultivating "positive" emotional attitudes and responses that may not arise spontaneously. As we discuss in detail in Chapter 6, deliberately cultivating loving-kindness, compassion, or gratitude toward people for whom we also feel anger or contempt can indeed strengthen these salutary states of mind. We need careful discernment to sense when we're using these practices as acts of avoidance because we have difficulty tolerating negative feelings, versus when we're using them to develop useful qualities of mind after fully experienced troubling emotions.

IT'S COMPLICATED, BUT WORTH IT

We've seen that bringing mindfulness into psychotherapy is, as the Dalai Lama (2009) suggested, "complicated." Human beings are multifaceted, and as a result no single practice or technique is going to be optimal for everyone at all times. The guidelines we've suggested in this chapter are just suggestions. Each therapist will need to discover, in the laboratory of the clinical hour, how various techniques affect different patients at different moments.

In the following pages, we examine in detail the many types of mindfulness practice described in this chapter. We present instructions for a wide range of techniques that you and your patients can try in different circumstances, along with clinical illustrations of how to apply them. Many of the practices we use most frequently are also available without charge online as reproducible patient handouts and as audio recordings at *www.sittingtogether.com*. Less frequently used meditation practices suited to the needs of particular individuals, along with guidelines for selecting practices for specific disorders and populations, can be found in the Appendix.

Our hope is that these practices will enliven your experience as a psychotherapist, while helping you and your patients to live richer, more rewarding lives.

CHAPTER TWO

Becoming a Mindful Therapist

Whatever you would make habitual, practice it; and if you would not make a thing habitual, do not practice it, but accustom yourself to something else.
—EPICTETUS (in Bartlett, 1980, p. 121)

The foundation for becoming more mindful human beings—and in the process, more mindful therapists—is our own mindfulness meditation practice. Without it, we may have an intellectual understanding of what mindfulness is about, but we won't be able to feel it in our bones. Nor will we be able to appreciate fully how it can transform the way we relate to the constantly changing, often highly charged phenomena in our outer and inner worlds.

That's why meditation teachers in all the major traditions are expected to develop and deepen their own practice before they can begin to teach others. It's also why instructors in programs such as mindfulness-based stress reduction (MBSR) and mindfulness-based cognitive therapy (MBCT) are required to learn and practice some form of mindfulness meditation. For the same reason, we believe those interested in practicing mindfulness-informed or mindfulness-based psychotherapy, who wish to do more than suggest informal mindfulness practices to patients, should begin by establishing their own meditation practice.

If you don't already have your own mindfulness practice, this chapter will help you get started. If you do, it will encourage you to expand and deepen it, and offer guidance for bringing mindfulness practice into your clinical work.

DO THERAPISTS BENEFIT FROM MINDFULNESS TRAINING?

A review of recent research shows that therapists and other health care professionals who practice mindfulness meditation enjoy a variety of benefits with no apparent negative effects (Escuriex & Labbé, 2011). The benefits include a decrease in perceived job stress, distress, and burnout (Galantino, Baime, Maguire, Szapary, & Farrar, 2005; Schenstrom, Ronnberg, & Bodlund, 2006; Shapiro, Astin, Bishop, & Cordova, 2005), as well as an increase in self-acceptance, self-compassion, satisfaction with life, and sense of well-being (Cohen-Katz et al., 2005; Schenstrom et al., 2006; Shapiro et al., 2005). What's more, participants reported improvements in their relationships with their patients, saying they felt better able to create a caring environment, had a greater capacity for empathy, and experienced an increased ability to be present in relationships without becoming reactive or defensive (Cohen-Katz et al., 2005; Pipe et al., 2009).

Therapist Effectiveness

Are therapists who practice mindfulness more effective in their work? Here, the research is less conclusive. One study (Grepmair et al., 2007) followed two groups of therapists in training, only one of which was given formal mindfulness training. Later, patients of both groups were surveyed. Patients of the therapists who received mindfulness training not only rated their experience in therapy significantly higher but also showed a greater reduction in symptoms. Another study (Greason & Cashwell, 2009) showed a connection between the mindfulness level of therapists in training and their ability to maintain attention and offer empathy. The authors conclude that mindfulness is a skill that enhances the therapeutic relationship. And in another study (Ryan, Safran, Deran, & Muran, 2012), patients of therapists with higher levels of dispositional mindfulness were more likely to see improvements in their interpersonal functioning, even if they didn't experience a reduction in symptoms. Other research, however, (Plummer, 2009; Stratton, 2006) shows no correlation between therapists' level of mindfulness and treatment results, and one study (Stanley et al., 2006) actually suggests that greater therapist mindfulness is associated with worse patient outcomes, perhaps related to decreased therapist fidelity to the treatment protocol, which in this case was a manualized approach. While the question of whether therapists' own mindfulness practice improves treatment outcomes has not yet been studied extensively experimentally, and more research is needed before clear conclusions can be drawn, we and many other therapists who practice mindfulness regularly believe it enhances therapeutic effectiveness.

Mindfulness and Therapeutic Presence

When we practice mindfulness, we repeatedly bring attention to our experience in the present moment. Again and again we let go of our ruminations about the past or anxieties about the future and return our attention to what is happening *right now*. We begin by focusing on relatively simple objects, such as the sensations of the breath entering the nostrils or the feet touching the floor. Gradually, as we develop the skill, we're able to focus on more complex objects, such as a patient sitting in front of us describing a painful memory from high school. This ability to be mindful, not stuck in the past or leaning into the future, but open to and accepting of whatever is emerging from moment to moment, is one definition of *presence*. Another is offered by psychologist and meditation teacher Tara Brach (2012), who suggests that presence is "the felt sense of wakefulness, openness, and tenderness that arises when we are fully here and now with our experience" (p. 12).

In many ways, mindfulness and presence are synonymous. But mindfulness also refers to the process of training the mind to be and stay present. Psychiatrist Daniel Siegel (2010a) discusses how "mindful awareness training" leads to presence:

> In every sense of the term *mindful*—being conscientious and intentional in what we do, being open and creative with possibilities or being aware of the present moment without grasping onto judgments—being mindful is a state of awareness that enables us to be flexible and receptive and to have presence. (p. 1)

Siegel further outlines a model that describes how this presence can help create more secure, empathic therapeutic relationships. He explains how presence leads to *attunement*—our ability to put aside personal preoccupations and take in the essence of our patient's experience. Attunement, in turn, results in *resonance*, a state in which two otherwise separate entities, therapist and patient, become one functional whole. Resonance is "how we feel 'felt,' and this is how two individuals become a 'we'" (D. J. Siegel, 2010a, p. 55). The combination of presence, attunement, and resonance allows the patient to develop a sense of safety and trust, conditions that facilitate positive change.

Psychologist Thomas Bien (2006) describes another way that mindfulness increases our capacity to be present, in turn improving our ability to listen deeply. In Bien's view, being fully present and listening deeply enables us to transform the psychotherapeutic hour into a profound, even spiritual encounter that fosters a sense of interconnection that allows the patient to heal and grow.

As we explore in the next chapter, mindfulness also helps us stay present by enhancing our capacity to tolerate the often powerful reactions we feel as we sit and listen to a patient (broadly described in psychoanalytic traditions as countertransference). For example, we can learn not to act on narcissistic impulses, such as the need to make an insightful comment in order to feel helpful or be admired. Or we can learn to step back, see our thoughts and feelings as just thoughts and feelings rather than facts, and instead of getting lost in them, we can redirect our attention back to the patient and to the inner and outer experience that is unfolding in the present moment.

Of course, reading about mindfulness is like reading about a wonderful new dish on a restaurant's menu. It may whet our appetites, but we can't really experience it until we taste it ourselves. And to taste some of the benefits of mindfulness, we need to practice.

GETTING STARTED: THE BASICS

Forms of Practice

As discussed in Chapter 1, mindfulness practice takes three basic forms. In *informal* practice, the practitioner brings conscious attention to the activities of daily life, such as washing the dishes, making the bed, or drinking a cup of tea. *Formal* practice, on the other hand, requires the practitioner to devote a regular block of time, put aside the activities of daily life and other distractions, and focus exclusively on developing one or more of the core mindfulness skills: concentration, open monitoring, and acceptance. (Detailed instructions for cultivating these skills are presented in Chapters 4–7.) In *intensive* practice, the practitioner goes to a retreat center or other protected environment to practice intensively for a day, a week, or even longer.

So where do you begin? If you're like most people, the easiest place to start is with informal practice since it requires no extra investment of time. Here's a simple practice you can start using right away.

WALKING TO THE WAITING ROOM MEDITATION

- Before you greet your next patient, form the intention to stay present in your body as best you can. Take one or two conscious breaths, letting go of any leftover feelings from your last session on the outbreath. Feel the sensations in the body as it contacts the floor and chair.

- As you get up, bring awareness to the various physical sensations that occur as the body changes position from sitting to standing.

- As you begin to walk, feel the contact of the feet against the floor. When reaching for the doorknob, notice how it feels in the hand. When you step out into the hallway, sense if the air feels or smells any different than it did in your office.

- Should thoughts and feelings appear, allow them to arise and pass as best you can, bringing your attention back to momentary physical sensations.

- Continue to feel the feet touching the floor as you walk down the hall.

- When you see your patient and say hello, be aware of the sensations in your throat, hear the sound your voice makes, and be open to whatever this other human being is bringing to the encounter. See if you can remain mindful during the session.

This is just one example of an informal mindfulness practice. You'll find others later in this chapter and throughout the rest of the book. These practices can help create some continuity of mindfulness throughout the day and are even more effective when they're used in conjunction with formal practice.

TAKING THE NEXT STEP

Although informal practice is a good place to start and an important way to cultivate mindfulness in daily life, it usually does not offer the opportunity to go deep enough to tap fully into the transformative power of mindfulness. In order to do that, most people also have to devote at least some time each day to formal practice.

Formal meditation instruction can be found throughout this book, as well as in many meditation centers, audio programs, websites, and other locations (see the Resources for listings).

If you really want to deepen your practice, there's no better way than taking the time for an extended retreat. As discussed earlier, going on retreat gives you a chance to be removed from the distractions and responsibilities of daily life and free from ordinary social conventions such as eye contact and conversation. In silence, the seemingly endless chattering of the mind can slow down to a much greater degree than it can in daily life, and the experience of mindfulness can become more continuous. As a result, insights can emerge about one's own personal history, the larger reality we all share, and how the mind creates suffering for itself. This is why retreats are valued in so many spiritual traditions and why instructors in mindfulness-based programs such as MBSR and MBCT are required to complete a weeklong silent retreat as part of their training. (For more information about retreats, see Chapter 10 and the Resources.)

Making the Commitment to Practice

Learning formal mindfulness practice is relatively simple, but keeping our practice going is not. Many challenges can arise once we decide to meditate regularly. It's easy to get frustrated, to start thinking we're not doing it right, and to start wondering if it's really worth the trouble. We can also get so preoccupied with the demands of daily life that we don't make the time to practice consistently, or we may stop altogether.

That's where commitment comes in. Expecting quick, clear results is one of the biggest problems we encounter. And who can blame us? We may have read about research showing that regular meditation practice has positive effects on brain structure and functioning (Davidson, 2004; Lazar et al., 2005; Hölzel et al., 2008), improves affect regulation (Ramel, Goldin, Carmona, & McQuaid, 2004), protects against depression (Kuyken et al., 2008; Godfrin & van Heeringen, 2010), reduces anxiety (McKim, 2008; Farb et al., 2010), and provides a host of other psychological and physiological benefits (see Germer, Siegel, & Fulton, 2013, for comprehensive reviews). What we may not have read is that the changes are often subtle and gradual. They're generally noticed over time, in retrospect. In fact, most studies look at people who have been practicing daily formal meditation for at least 8 to 10 weeks, and sometimes much longer.

We mentioned earlier how cultivating mindfulness is a bit like developing physical fitness, in that we can take it up with different levels of intensity. The analogy also holds in another way: Sometimes it can be challenging to get into an exercise routine, as on some days a workout may be quite difficult, whereas on other days the same workout feels relatively effortless. But whether workouts are easy or challenging, we feel confident that the body is becoming more fit every time we do physical exercise. So too with mindfulness—whether the practice feels easy or hard, whether we find the mind frisky or calm, each moment of practice helps to cultivate a little more mindfulness.

So it's important to keep going, and not judge our practice too soon. If you're just starting, commit to practicing for at least 8 weeks before you come to any conclusions. Just keep sitting without evaluating how you're doing or expecting any particular results. Then, after the 8 weeks, you can look back and decide whether anything has changed, and whether it's worth continuing.

Eight Ways to Maintain a Mindfulness Practice

How do you stay motivated in the face of uncertainty, doubt, and the demands of patients, family, and friends—not to mention your own mind? Here are some tips you might find useful.

1. *Make it a habit.* Like brushing your teeth, make meditation part of your daily routine. Decide which time of day works best for you—first thing in the morning or sometime in the evening (or both) are usually good choices—and build that time into your schedule. Then don't even think about it. Most important, don't worry about whether you feel like it. As they used to say in the Nike ads, just do it.

2. *Not too long or too short.* Choose a length of time for formal practice that's long enough to allow the mind to begin to settle, but not so long that you won't be able to make it a regular part of your life. For most people, somewhere between 15 and 45 minutes a day is about right. But if all you can manage is 5 or 10 minutes, that's better than nothing. And it's probably wise to start small and gradually lengthen the amount of time as you gain confidence and experience.

3. *Create a sacred space.* You may not have the luxury of being able to set aside an entire room for sitting quietly, as some practitioners do. But if at all possible, create a space for meditation in the corner of your bedroom, living room, or office. Set it up so that you don't have to re-create it each time you want to practice, so that you can just sit down and begin. If you wish, decorate the space with objects and images that inspire you.

4. *Find your seat.* If your practice involves sitting, as most formal mindfulness practices do, be sure to sit in a way that allows you to remain upright, but relaxed and comfortable at the same time. The right posture encourages wakefulness, instills a sense of dignity, and facilitates the smooth flow of the breath from the nose through the trachea to the lungs. In traditional Buddhist communities, practitioners typically sit on either a small cushion, known as a *zafu*, or a meditation bench. But a straight-back chair is also fine. You might want to experiment with all three, or even alternate among them, depending on how your body feels (see the following box for more detailed posture instructions).

5. *Seek other forms of support.* Getting guidance from a qualified meditation teacher, either in person or through books and audio recordings, can be invaluable. Sitting together with a friend or in a community of like-minded people can also help sustain and enliven your practice through its inevitable ups and downs.

6. *Suspend judgment.* As mentioned earlier, having unreasonable expectations and judging yourself against them will inevitably lead to frustration. Instead, remember that it's not about getting anywhere special, but about coming back again and again to where you already are.

7. *Be gentle but persistent.* Meditation requires effort, but trying too hard can be counterproductive. Instead, seek the Middle Way, which the Buddha described with a metaphor about the strings of a lute: In order to produce music, they must be neither too tight nor too loose. Another way to think of this is to be gentle with yourself, but keep going.

8. *Remember your intention.* Why did you decide to practice in the first place? To find peace of mind? To be more present for your patients, your partner, your friends, yourself? To bring more wisdom and compassion into the world? Keeping your highest intention in mind can be a powerful source of motivation, particularly when you're feeling lost, confused, or discouraged.

Finding an Optimal Physical Posture for Meditation

If you choose to sit up, you can use a chair, a meditation cushion, or a meditation bench. If using a chair, find one that allows you to sit comfortably with a more or less straight spine. This posture helps us pay attention—having a straight spine increases alertness. You can use the back of the chair for support if you like, or sit a bit forward, finding a balanced position in which your spine supports itself.

If using a meditation cushion, place the cushion on a folded blanket or carpet to create a soft surface on which to sit cross-legged. The cushion needs to be tall enough so that your knees can touch the floor, forming a stable triangle between your two knees on the ground and your buttocks on the cushion. You can place one foot on top of the opposite ankle or calf or simply allow both feet to lie on the floor, one just in front of the other, without actually crossing them. If you find your legs or feet becoming numb ("falling asleep"), try adding another cushion or folded blanket to sit a bit higher. The idea is to find a posture that feels comfortable and stable with a relaxed, yet erect spine.

If using a meditation bench, place it on a folded blanket or carpet. Begin by kneeling, with your knees, shins, and feet against the ground. Then place the bench under you so that it supports your buttocks and most of your weight. You may also want to put a cushion or folded blanket on top of the bench to give yourself more height and padding. Here, too, the idea is to find a posture that feels comfortable and stable with a more or less straight spine.

Regardless of how you choose to sit, you may find it helpful to imagine that a string is attached to the top of your head, pulling you gently toward the ceiling or sky, lengthening your spine. Next gently rock your head forward and back and from side to side to find a position where it balances naturally. The idea is to arrive at a relaxed yet dignified and alert posture. You can rest your hands comfortably on your thighs or knees to add to a sense of stability. Try not to use your arms to support your torso or to keep from falling back-ward, as this creates a lot of tension.

While meditation is not really a physical exercise, it will be useful to try to remain as still as possible while meditating. If an urge arises to scratch an itch or adjust your position, experiment with just observing the urge without acting on it. While you don't have to be heroic or stoic about this, exercising some restraint with the urge to move will enhance your concentration. It will also illustrate an important principle about how the mind habitually reacts to discomfort—a principle at the heart of mindfulness practice.

Note. Adapted from R. D. Siegel (2010). Copyright 2010 by Ronald D. Siegel. Adapted by permission.

BRINGING MINDFULNESS INTO THE CONSULTING ROOM

Let's assume you've begun to establish a formal mindfulness practice and have made it a part of your life. How can you bring it more directly into your clinical work—not only by teaching it to patients, which is discussed in Chapters 4 through 7, but also by embodying it yourself? There are three basic ways: (1) creating the right conditions for mindfulness in your work, (2) finding the time for formal practice during the workday, and (3) building informal practices into your day.

Creating the Conditions for Mindfulness

Mindfulness is more likely to arise when certain conditions are present, conditions that can be described by four related terms, all beginning with the letter *s: spaciousness, simplicity, single-mindedness,* and *slowing down.*

When we are mindful, there's a sense of *spaciousness* in which thoughts, feelings, and physical sensations can come and go more freely. By adding some *external* spaciousness to our day, we can put ourselves in a position to experience the *internal* spaciousness of mindfulness more easily and more often. One way to do this is to arrive in your office at least a few minutes earlier than you have to. This will give you a chance not only to tidy up the room and adjust the temperature and lighting but also to get grounded in the space, and perhaps even take a few mindful breaths before your first patient arrives. If possible, see if you can also build in some space between appointments and make space in your schedule for lunch and other breaks.

Years ago, one of us had the opportunity to interview Walt Frazier, the legendary National Basketball Association player who was famous for being able to keep his cool, both on and off the court. When asked what his secret was, Frazier replied that he never allowed himself to feel rushed, and that to set the proper tone, he always arrived at the arena before the other players on game days so that he could calmly prepare himself both physically and mentally for the contest ahead (personal communication, 1984). Preparing ourselves to participate in a series of intense therapeutic encounters with our patients is not so different. In order to do it well, in order to increase the chances that we'll be able to stay present and attuned, we need to give ourselves some time and space.

Simplicity is an attitude. It involves setting aside preoccupations with the past and worries about the future and coming back, again and again, to the here and now. It means letting go of everything we know about psychological theories and everything we think we know about our patient and meeting him or her in the freshness of *this* moment. Simplicity can also be reflected in our physical surroundings. By keeping our office relatively neat and uncluttered, we can create a sanctuary that makes it easier for our patients and ourselves to stay focused on the task at hand.

Closely related to simplicity is *single-mindedness,* which in this context means doing just one thing at a time, or *single-tasking.* Of course, when we're sitting with our patients, we do everything we can to make sure our sessions are not interrupted and our attention is not divided. But we can also try extending this approach to the rest of our day by avoiding multitasking as much as possible. So when we're talking on the phone, we're just talking on the phone. When we're writing a progress note, we're just writing a progress note. When we're eating our lunch, we're just eating our lunch. There's no need to be fanatical about this; inevitably, we will have to make exceptions. But if you'd like to be more single-minded during sessions, we suggest you try being more single-minded between sessions as well.

Finally, *slowing down* is a great aid to mindfulness. One of the best ways we can do this is by remembering to press the pause button—to simply pause and take a breath, especially when we're feeling confused or stirred up emotionally. Tara Brach (2003) sees the "sacred pause" as an opportunity to interrupt deeply conditioned, often destructive patterns of reactivity so that we can choose wiser, more skillful responses instead. Buddhist teacher Pema Chodron (2009) suggests that pausing is a powerful way to connect with "natural openness," which she describes as "the spaciousness of our skylike minds":

> Pausing is very helpful in this process. It creates a momentary contrast between being completely self-absorbed and being awake and present. You just stop for a few seconds, breathe deeply, and move on. (pp. 7–8)

To the developers of MBCT, pausing allows us to switch from the "doing mode" to the "being mode," so that we can stop running on automatic pilot and start acting with greater mindfulness as we care for ourselves and others (Segal, Williams, & Teasdale, 2002).

Formal Practices for the Clinical Day

If you can make the time, here are some brief formal mindfulness practices you might want to incorporate into your clinical day.

This first meditation can be done anytime but is particularly useful at the start of the clinical day. It is inspired by a meditation from Thomas Bien (2006) called "Becoming the Guru" (pp. 26–27). Not strictly a mindfulness exercise, it also includes visualization, a technique that is used in many spiritual traditions, especially when the purpose of the practice is the cultivation of positive qualities associated with mindfulness such as compassion, loving-kindness, and equanimity.

MERGING WITH THE SOURCE

- Sit in an upright but comfortable posture and slowly begin to bring attention to the breath. Sense the body expanding on the inbreath and contracting, or letting go, on the outbreath.

- Should you notice that the attention has wandered, as it may many times, gently put aside whatever took the attention away and bring it back to the sensations of breathing.

- Gradually narrow the focus of attention so that it is concentrated in the chest and upper back, the area surrounding the heart.

- While staying connected with the sensations of breathing around the heart, bring to mind a being who embodies the highest levels of wisdom and compassion. If you're religious or spiritually inclined, it could be the Buddha, Jesus Christ, Kwan Yin, Mother Teresa, or a figure from your own tradition or community. If you're of a more secular bent, it could be someone from history or mythology, or a beloved teacher, clinical supervisor, or mentor. It could even be your own higher self. Or instead of just one being, you could imagine a series of such beings standing around you in a circle, their eyes filled with wisdom and compassion.

- Now imagine a beam of light connecting your heart with the heart of this being or circle of beings. As you continue to breathe, feel yourself taking in their positive qualities and healing energy. See the light between your hearts beginning to intensify. Allow the distance between your hearts to shrink gradually until you have become one with the source.

- Sit quietly for a few more moments and imagine this supreme source of wisdom and compassion infusing your entire body from head to toe. Form an intention to remember that it is always there, and to bring it into your work with your patients, as best you can, throughout the rest of the day.

This next meditation takes just 1 to 5 minutes, depending on how much time you have, so it can usually be done between sessions or at other times during the day when you're feeling lost in the past or future and want to reconnect with the here and now. It is adapted from the "Three-Minute Breathing Space," an exercise developed as part of the MBCT program (Segal et al., 2002).

MINI-MINDFULNESS BREAK

- Sit in an upright position with feet flat on the ground. Allow the eyes to close or just look down a few feet in front of you without focusing on anything in particular. (You can also do this exercise standing or lying down if you prefer.)

- Bring awareness to the body/mind and acknowledge any strong sensations or energy you find. Briefly name the experience if you can (by saying to yourself something like "tightness in the lower back," "feeling anxious," or "thinking about something that was said in the last session"). As you note whatever it is you're experiencing, remember to be as objective and accepting of it as you possibly can be. The idea is simply to name what is happening, not to judge or analyze it.

- Redirect your awareness to the sensations of breathing, focusing on either the tip of the nose, the chest, or the abdomen, wherever you feel the breath most strongly. As best you can, make the breath sensations your exclusive object of attention, staying with them for at least three full inbreaths and three full outbreaths, longer if you have the time and inclination. When your attention wanders, put aside whatever caused it to wander and gently bring it back to the breath.

- Staying connected with the breath, gradually expand your field of awareness to include the whole body, so there's an awareness of the breath together with sensations elsewhere.

- Continue expanding the field of awareness by adding sounds and the experience of hearing. Just notice sounds as they arise and pass away.

- Open the eyes, look around, and bring awareness to the next thing you see, think, feel, say, or do.

Every therapist knows the feeling. It's 15 minutes past the hour and your patient hasn't shown up. Perhaps you've called and left a message. Or maybe you're just waiting and wondering: Was there a last-minute emergency? Was there a misunderstanding about the appointment time? Did he or she just forget? Or did something come up during the last session that's making it difficult for him or her to return? Maybe my patient is dropping out of treatment and I'll never hear from him or her again. In a situation like this, the mind can make up a lot of stories to explain the unknown.

Since there's nothing you can do about it now, how might you use this unexpected gift of 45 extra minutes in the middle of your day? Of course, you could catch up with paperwork, make phone calls, surf the Web, or read a few pages in that novel you started yesterday. But before tackling your to-do list, you might want to try the following meditation, which is designed to cultivate mindfulness and compassion in the face of uncertainty and doubt:

NO-SHOW MEDITATION

- Sit quietly, close your eyes, and bring awareness to any thoughts appearing in the mind. If you think you know why your patient hasn't shown up, remind yourself that this is just a thought, a best guess, and consider other possible explanations. If you realize that you really don't know, then see if you can simply sit with the uncertainty.

- Briefly acknowledge any feelings that might be arising. Perhaps you're feeling annoyed, hurt, confused, worried, anxious, or lonely. Instead of feeding the feelings with more thinking, see if you can locate them in your body and breathe with them or into them. Ask yourself: Can I make space for these difficult thoughts and feelings?

- As best you can, put the thoughts aside and give your full attention to physical sensations. If you've located a spot in your body that seems to be holding the experience—a knot in your stomach or tightness in your chest, for example— you may choose to focus on that. Or you may prefer to concentrate on the touch points (where the body touches the chair, floor, or itself), the body as a whole, or the sensations of breathing. For at least a few minutes, use these physical sensations as an anchor, remembering to keep coming back to them whenever you notice your attention has wandered.

- While staying in touch with these sensations, begin sending yourself loving-kindness by slowly and silently repeating phrases such as the following: *May I be safe and protected from inner and outer harm. May I have ease of mind. May I have comfort of heart. May I be free from all forms of suffering.* (For more on loving-kindness practice, see Chapter 6.)

- After a while, shift focus by bringing to mind an image or felt sense of your patient. Then begin extending loving-kindness to him or her: *May you be safe and protected from inner and outer harm. May you have ease of mind. May you have comfort of heart. May you be free from all forms of suffering.*
- Finally, bring to mind all beings who are currently separated from someone they care about. This group may include other therapists and patients, parents who are separated from their children, friends separated from friends, lovers separated from their beloved: *May we be safe and protected from inner and outer harm. May we have ease of mind. May we have comfort of heart. May we be free from all forms of suffering.*
- Before going on with your day, spend some time simply breathing and being with whatever sensations in the body are most vivid. See if you can carry a sense of loving-kindness and compassion into your next activity.

More Informal Practices for the Clinical Day

You might be thinking that you're just too busy to incorporate much formal mindfulness practice into your clinical day. And that might be true. But even in the busiest settings on the most hectic days, there are always opportunities to practice informally. All you have to do is look for little spaces in the midst of the busyness and then remember to be mindful. The *Walking to the Waiting Room Meditation* described previously in this chapter is one possibility. But there are many more.

For example, as you develop your meditation practice, you'll become more and more familiar with your anchors—places to which you return your attention when the mind has wandered. Returning to the anchor is like coming home after you've been lost. It offers a sense of safety and comfort. It can also be a valuable informal practice when you're in a challenging clinical situation.

Let's say you're sitting with a patient who's reciting a litany of familiar self-criticisms, or who's angry about a comment you've made, or who confesses he or she has been thinking about suicide. You find yourself feeling anxious, afraid, frustrated, annoyed, and/or confused. You notice yourself leaning forward in your seat. You wonder if you're up to the challenge, if you can come up with something useful to say. Before speaking, you could try this:

RETURNING TO THE ANCHOR

- Instead of thinking about what to say, return to an anchor, if only for a few seconds. Take a conscious breath or two. Feel the contact of the body against the chair. Hear the background hum of the ventilation system or the car passing outside.
- If you have a well-established loving-kindness or compassion practice, you can also return to the phrases as an anchor.

Connecting with an anchor gives you a chance to come back into the present moment, to dispel the clouds of doubt and confusion, and to allow your innate wisdom and compassion to inform whatever you say or do next.

Psychologist and meditation teacher Sylvia Boorstein (2011a) says she often lets the loving-kindness or compassion phrases play in the back of her mind "like a little metronome" that helps her stay balanced during difficult clinical encounters: "As soon as I'm balanced, I'm back in the room . . . completely. Then my own mind regains its own wisdom . . . and actually what arises then is my natural compassion" (p. 7).

More than many other professionals, psychotherapists, especially those in private practice, often dine alone during their work hours, squeezing in a quick meal or snack between appointments. This can also be a wonderful opportunity to cultivate mindfulness. Here are a few suggestions:

MINDFUL MEAL BREAKS

- Set aside your laptop, smartphone, paperwork, reading material, and other distractions.
- Look at your food and reflect briefly on all the natural and human forces that came together in order to produce it and make it available to you.
- Take in the aroma of your food before you eat it.
- When you do take a bite, give your full attention to the experience. Notice the texture, the flavor, and any reactions that might be occurring in your body and mind.
- If you have the time, chew more slowly than usual and pause briefly between bites.
- When you're done, resolve to use the energy this food has

given you to stay more awake and present for yourself and your patients during the rest of the day.

(See Chapter 6 for more details about an eating meditation.)

Answering the phone is another common, work-related activity you can use as an informal mindfulness practice. All you have to do is remember to pay attention:

ANSWERING THE PHONE

- When the phone rings, really listen to the sound before you make any move to answer the call.
- When you pick up the phone, feel its weight, texture, temperature, and other physical properties.
- If you check the caller ID, notice any thoughts and feelings that appear, whether or not you recognize the name and number.
- As the conversation begins, be aware of speaking and listening. Hear the sound of your own voice. Listen to the sound of the caller's voice. Monitor any reactions that arise, and if you find yourself getting caught up in them, stay connected with your body or some other anchor.
- When the call ends, pause for a moment or two and bring attention back to the body, paying particular attention to any areas of tightness or tension. Breathe into these areas, and see if it's possible to make space for the sensations there before going on with your day.

WHAT TO DO WHEN YOU'RE FEELING DISCOURAGED

Developing our own meditation practice can have innumerable benefits for us personally and professionally. It does not always go smoothly, however. Feeling discouraged is an inevitable part of the process, especially if we tend to have high expectations. Whenever you (or your patients) feel like quitting, it can be helpful to remember the following points:

- *Patience is required.* The changes that take place during meditation are subtle and gradual. Often it seems like nothing is happening.

But it is. Many studies have shown measurable improvements, including changes in brain functioning and objective performance, in people who have practiced consistently for 8 to 10 weeks.

- *The benefits are cumulative.* When you practice meditation, you are rewiring responses to physical and emotional experiences that have been conditioned for as long as you've been alive. This doesn't happen overnight. Most of the changes and benefits can only be noticed over time, in retrospect.

- *Pay attention to the discouragement.* Can you be mindful of the discouragement and of related states such as boredom and restlessness? Watch them closely. Get curious about them. How do you actually experience them? Try breaking them down into their components: thoughts, feelings, and physical sensations.

- *Be kind.* Practice isn't easy. It is in the nature of the mind to wander. So each time you notice that the mind has wandered, it's not a problem. In fact, you should congratulate yourself because you're already back on track. If the mind wanders a thousand times, you simply bring it back a thousand times. That's what practice is all about.

- *Don't compare.* All you can do is practice to the best of your ability. Don't compare yourself with anyone else or to where you think you should be. Just be where you are, and let that be enough.

MOVING BEYOND US

The suggestions and exercises in this chapter are primarily geared toward developing mindfulness in ourselves. And for most of us, that is the best place to start. In the next chapter, we explore the next logical step for the mindfulness-oriented clinician: How to cultivate mindfulness in our relationships with our patients, increasing our levels of interpersonal attunement and resonance along the way, so that each 50-minute hour can become a "two-person meditation" (Epstein, 2008).

CHAPTER THREE

Cultivating Mindfulness
in the Therapeutic Relationship

To sense the client's private world as if it were your own—
but without ever losing the "as if" quality—this is empathy,
and this seems essential to therapy.
                                        —CARL ROGERS (1961, p. 284)

Lester Luborsky, the pioneering psychotherapy outcomes researcher, is famous for advancing the "Dodo Bird hypothesis." After years of compiling meta-analytic studies, he and his colleagues concluded that the contest for the most effective form of psychotherapy had finally been settled. As the Dodo Bird declared at the finish of a race in *Alice in Wonderland*, "Everybody has won and all must have prizes" (Luborsky, Singer, & Luborsky, 1975). While subsequent researchers have argued vigorously for and against this position, there are compelling data that a remarkably wide range of therapies are indeed effective for a great many disorders. A great deal of data also suggest that the particular technique employed by a psychotherapist is often less important than "common factors," such as the strength of the therapeutic alliance, in predicting outcome (Duncan & Miller, 2000; Fulton, 2013;

Hatcher, 2010; Horvath, Del Re, Flückiger, & Symonds, 2011; Stiles, 2009; Tryon & Winograd, 2011).

Although many mindfulness-based treatments show promise in outcome studies, of at least equal importance is the potential of mindfulness practices to improve the quality of therapy relationships generally. Chapter 2 presents preliminary evidence that the therapist's own mindfulness practice can enhance his or her emotional attunement and therapeutic presence. In this chapter, we offer suggestions as to how we can use mindfulness practices to deepen our therapeutic alliances, and how we might best maintain these alliances when introducing mindfulness practices to our patients.

DEEPENING THERAPEUTIC PRESENCE

Current studies suggest that in successful treatment alliances, therapists are perceived to be warm, empathic, understanding, and accepting, approaching their patients with an open, collaborative attitude (Norcross & Wampold, 2011). Many years earlier, Freud (1912) suggested that we strive to cultivate "evenly hovering attention" in which the therapist "has simply to listen and not to trouble to keep in mind anything in particular" (pp. 111–112). But neither Freud nor modern researchers indicate how we might cultivate these abilities. Mindfulness practices may provide a method.

Focused Attention

A foundational skill in mindfulness practices is concentration, or focused attention (see Chapters 1 and 4). Simply by bringing our awareness repeatedly to an object of attention, whether the breath, the soles of our feet touching the ground, or sounds of nature, we strengthen our capacity to focus. This ability can be enormously useful in the therapy hour, where many factors can cause the mind to wander. The content of the session might threaten us, so our attention drifts defensively; an outside worry or concern may pull at our attention; our patient might become disengaged, making his or her words less interesting; or perhaps we just get tired, drawing our attention toward REM sleep. Under all of these circumstances, developing concentration can help us to remain focused.

Without mindfulness training, we typically try to maintain our attention by turning up the volume, increasing the intensity of an experience in order to keep it "interesting." Through mindfulness practice, we instead learn to turn up our attention, to practice presence independent of content, developing what Karen Horney (1952/1998, p. 36) called "wholehearted" attention (see also Morgan, Morgan, & Germer, 2013).

Here is a simple exercise you can try with a colleague that can provide insight into the nature of our attention during sessions and what contributes to our mind wandering.

WHAT BRINGS YOU AWAY?

- Sit in an upright but comfortable posture facing your partner. Begin by both closing your eyes, bringing attention to the breath. Sense the body expanding on the inbreath and contracting, or letting go, on the outbreath.

- Should you notice that the attention has wandered, gently let go of whatever took the attention away and bring it back to the sensations of breathing.

- After a few minutes, open your eyes. Decide who will begin as the speaker, and who as the listener.

- The listener's job is to *just listen*. This means refraining from nodding, from smiling, from telling your partner that you understand his or her feelings. Just take in the amazing audiovisual experience of your partner's presence.

- The speaker's job is to muse aloud about the following question: *What brings you away from being fully present in your work?* Try to say whatever comes to mind without censorship.

- Have the speaker speak, and the listener listen, for about 2 minutes.

- Next, switch roles; the listener becomes the speaker, and the speaker becomes the listener. Repeat the exercise for about 2 minutes.

- Discuss with your partner what you each noticed being the listener, and what you each noticed being the speaker.

Therapists typically report a variety of reactions to this exercise. As listeners, most find that it is initially difficult to refrain from the usual demonstrations of understanding—nodding, smiling, or otherwise attempting to show the other person that we're listening. Sometimes this urge to communicate dominates the listener's awareness and makes it difficult to focus, but sometimes the restraint frees the listener to really listen, unburdened of the need to prove to the speaker that he or she is being heard.

As speakers, some therapists find that the listener's lack of nodding or otherwise affirming that they're being heard is challenging—it makes them feel abandoned. Others find that the open space created by the listener *just listening* frees them to really explore their feelings. Either way, therapists often gain insight into what brings their attention away during their work.

We're not suggesting that therapists adopt this *just listening* stance, not responding demonstratively to patients. But trying this exercise with a colleague can help us to be more mindful of what we do automatically. An experienced therapist can nod, ask for clarifications or elaborations, and appear to demonstrate understanding, all while planning a 12-course meal. Noticing our well-practiced responses, along with what brings our attention away, can help us to be more present in our work.

Affect Tolerance

Of the many factors that interfere with our attention during therapy, one of the most challenging is the arousal of powerful, painful feelings. While occasionally our patients share their good fortune with us, more often they discuss difficult experiences such as illness, loss, failure, and disappointment. Unless we're very good at denial, we notice that our patients' misfortunes could readily befall us or our loved ones. And sometimes that thought is hard to bear.

Mindfulness practices can be powerful tools to increase our affect tolerance, allowing us to remain attentive when bearing witness to pain. Remaining attentive is essential for maintaining a strong therapeutic alliance because our patients typically will express only those feelings that they feel we can tolerate hearing. If some emotions are too raw or difficult for us to tolerate, our patients will notice that, and typically back away from exploring them. On the other hand, if we are able to *be with* a fuller range of experiences, this will help our patients to do the same. One of us was taught this by a patient early in his career:

CLINICAL ILLUSTRATION: BEING WITH PAINFUL FEELINGS

Jerry was a depressed young man who was convinced that he had no possibility of happiness, no chance of finding friends or love. Week after week he told me of his hopeless situation, and I made feeble attempts to help. I suggested different ways to handle interactions, reasons why his situation might improve some day. I often left sessions quite depressed myself, thinking, "I was a good student, I could have gone into so many fields, this is clearly not my calling." Every once in a while, however, after a particularly depressing session, Jerry would return the next week looking a little brighter. He even occasionally suggested that our previous session was a bit helpful. I would think, "To *you* maybe—it just made me depressed."

Gradually I learned a lesson: If I could accompany Jerry into his darkest places and feel in myself some of the stuckness and helplessness he felt, he'd feel a little less alone, a little more understood, a little more hopeful.*

How can we use mindfulness practices to develop this sort of affect tolerance? There are two pathways that complement each other: practicing being with discomfort and observing the impersonal nature of feelings.

Practicing Being with Discomfort

One way to increase our affect tolerance is to practice restraint during formal meditation practice.

BEING WITH DISCOMFORT

- Start by sitting comfortably, assuming a posture of dignity with your back straight, your spine relaxed but not rigid, eyes either softly open or closed.
- If all is going well, you'll find that you're already breathing. Simply notice the sensations of your breath.
- See where you feel your breath most strongly. It may be at the nostrils, at the chest, or in the belly. Allow yourself to feel the sensations of each inhalation and exhalation.

*Adapted from R. D. Siegel (2012). Copyright 2012 by The Guilford Press. Adapted by permission.

- If your mind wanders, no problem. Gently and lovingly bring your attention back to the breath.

- After following the breath for about 10 to 15 minutes, see if you can locate any discomfort in the body—perhaps an ache, or an itch.

- Instead of automatically scratching the itch or shifting posture to relieve the ache, allow the breath to be in the background and bring your full attention to the discomfort. Notice its texture, and how it changes from moment to moment.

- Stay with the sensations of discomfort as long as you can. If they become overwhelming, feel free to move, but first try the experiment of just staying with them for a while.

- After attending to the discomfort for several minutes, return your attention to the sensations of the breath.

Many people are surprised by what happens when they bring attention to physical discomfort in this way. Often they notice that pain sensations are not solid, but pulse and change from moment to moment. Sometimes they pass completely without any special action on our part.

By practicing being with discomfort during this sort of concentration exercise, we gradually become better able to tolerate pain of all sorts, including the pain of difficult emotions.

Not My Emotion, But the Emotion

Perhaps the most profound insight that can come from mindfulness practice is the discovery that "I" don't exist. Of course the body is here, others know us by our name, and we have an address and a Social Security number. But what we find in mindfulness practice is that our consciousness consists of an ever-changing flow of experience. Thoughts, feelings, and sensations arise and pass, but we never encounter the little homunculus—the little man or woman inside that's "me." There is no enduring, discrete self to be found. Rather, we just find this unfolding experience, regularly narrated by the words of the thought stream. We discover, as mentioned in Chapter 1, the fact of *anatta* or no-self—that we are "an orchestra without a conductor."

Although this notion can sound esoteric, experiencing no-self can enhance therapeutic presence by increasing our ability to be with intense feeling. Let's consider again the situation mentioned in Chapter 1 in which someone hurts our feelings. We might think, "I can't believe you did this to me after all that I've done for you." This thought would be followed by an uptick in angry emotions, which in turn would trigger more angry thoughts, increasing the intensity and duration of the episode (Farb et al., 2007).

How might this look through the experience of no-self revealed in mindfulness practice? We might notice muscles tensing in the neck and back, the heart beating more quickly, and perhaps images of confronting the person who upset us dancing through our mind. We would experience anger as a cognitive scientist might describe it: the co-arising of bodily sensations with a verbal narrative and visual imagery. Instead of the experience being about "my" anger (or "my" fear, pain, joy, etc.), it would be about "the" impersonal sensations, thoughts, and images arising. By not getting so caught in thoughts about "me" (and "you"), we'd be able to bear the emotion at much higher levels—to allow waves of emotion to arise and pass more freely. And, as we've seen, being able to stay with difficult feelings can be essential to maintaining an effective therapeutic alliance.

We can enhance our ability to abide and even embrace difficult affect in sessions by formally practicing being with emotions outside of the clinical hour. Here is an exercise that can help us do this.

EMBRACING EMOTIONS THAT ARISE IN THERAPY

- Start by sitting comfortably, assuming a posture of dignity with your back straight, your spine relaxed but not rigid, eyes either softly open or closed.
- Simply notice the sensations of the breath, wherever you feel them most strongly—perhaps at the tip of the nostrils or in the rising and falling of the abdomen.
- If your mind wanders, no problem. Gently and lovingly bring your attention back to the breath.
- After following the breath for a few minutes, recall a moment during a therapy session when you felt a strong emotion arise, perhaps some sadness, anger, or fear.
- See if you can feel a bit of that emotion now, noticing how it feels in the body.
- Next see if you can intensify the emotion, either by bringing your attention to it more fully, by re-imagining the therapy

session in which it first arose, or perhaps by generating
another thought or memory that will reinforce it.

- Now stay with the moment-to-moment experience of the
  emotion. Note the sensations in the throat, eyes, chest, belly,
  or wherever they arise. Notice what thoughts or images
  accompany the sensations. Try to stay with the experience for
  several minutes.

- After attending to the emotion in the body, return your
  attention to the sensations of the breath. Sit quietly for
  another few minutes, then open your eyes and return to your
  day.

The Zen tradition uses a metaphor to describe how these practices transform the mind: If I were to dissolve a tablespoon of salt in a glass of water and try to drink it, I'd have difficulty—the water would be unpalatably salty. But if I were to take that same tablespoon of salt and dissolve it into a clear, clean pond, I'd have no difficulty at all taking a sip. Mindfulness practices gradually transform the mind into such a clear pond, a mind that can accept whatever comes its way.

Zen tradition also includes a disturbing but moving story that illustrates the power of these practices to strengthen the mind and cultivate equanimity. This version is adapted from R. D. Siegel (2010):

One day in ancient Japan, a cruel, sadistic general rode into town with his army. His men immediately set about stealing whatever they could and wreaking havoc. They raped women, killed children, burned down houses, and destroyed crops. When the general caught wind that the people revered their Zen master, intent on fully vanquishing the population, he set out to kill him, too.

The general galloped his horse up the hill on the edge of town and rode right into the main hall of the Zen temple. There, meditating on a cushion, was a little old man. The general brought his horse up next to him and held his bloody sword over the man's head. The man looked up. "Don't you realize I could run you through with this sword without blinking an eye?" said the general. "Don't you realize I could be run through with that sword without blinking an eye?" said the Zen master. At this point the general became disoriented, bowed, and left town.

Now this isn't always going to work as a military intervention. But it gives a flavor of the courage and flexibility that mindfulness practice can cultivate. Having even a little of this courage can help us to stay more fully with our patients' experience, however difficult it may be.

GETTING OUT OF THE WAY

Another way that glimpsing *anatta*, or no-self, can support the therapeutic alliance is by helping therapists to let go of narcissistic preoccupations. As part of a project researching the role of wisdom in psychotherapy, one of us surveyed experienced therapists and asked, "What gets in the way of your acting wisely as a clinician?" A particularly wise respondent answered succinctly, "Me!"

Indeed, most practitioner errors that weaken the therapeutic alliance involve our narcissistic concerns—our wishes to be seen a certain way by our patients and colleagues. The universal human desire to be seen favorably by others (Gilbert, 2009a) can make us fake it when we forget what happened in last week's session, don't know as much as we think we should about a particular treatment or disorder, confuse the names of medications, or become sleepy or distracted during therapy. If we had fewer concerns about how we look to ourselves and others, we would be free to respond more skillfully and authentically to such lapses. Ironically, caring less about appearing competent allows us actually to *be* more competent.

Here's a little exercise that can help us recognize how narcissistic preoccupations might be getting in the way of our therapeutic alliances.

NOT WORRYING ABOUT ME

- Start by sitting comfortably, assuming a posture of dignity with your back straight, your spine relaxed but not rigid, eyes either softly open or closed.

- Simply notice the sensations of your breath, wherever you feel them most strongly.

- If your mind wanders, no problem. Gently and lovingly bring your attention back to the breath for a few minutes.

- Now imagine what a day at work would be like if you no longer had concerns about earning a living, being liked or respected by patients or colleagues, or thinking of yourself as professionally competent. How might you dress? What might you do differently? Reflect on your last several sessions and imagine how they might have unfolded.

- After reflecting on those sessions, return your attention to the sensations of the breath. Sit quietly for another few minutes, then open your eyes. As you return to your day, continue to notice the effects of your concerns for how you appear to yourself and others.

Befriending Our Shadow

Another way that mindfulness practice can enrich our therapeutic alliances is by illuminating how we construct our identities. Carl Jung pointed out that we tend to identify with some of our attributes as "me" and see others as definitely "not me." Our *personas* are made up of qualities we think of as "me," whereas those we think of as "not me" cluster unconsciously into what Jung (1938) called the *shadow*. So, if I like to think of myself as an intelligent, compassionate, generous person, I'm going to have difficulty whenever I notice my stupid, unfeeling, selfish shadow. Dividing our attributes into "me" and "not me" in this way can interfere with our capacity to form therapeutic alliances. Whenever something happens in therapy that highlights our shadow (e.g., our self-preoccupation, confusion, inattention, or ignorance), we tend to become defensive. Rejecting aspects of ourselves also makes us react negatively to our patients whenever they seem to share our disavowed qualities.

When we see that there is no separate enduring self, but rather just an unbroken flow of changing moments, we become less compelled to seek experiences that reinforce a particular view of ourselves. We come to appreciate that mindfulness practice is not a path to perfection but a path to wholeness (Brach, 2003). As we see our mind construct a "self" by identifying with some contents and rejecting others, we can better embrace all of our experiences. This can help us be less judgmental and more flexible in our responses to our patients.

A simple exercise can help us to become more conscious of the elements in our professional personas and shadows.

FINDING OUR PROFESSIONAL SHADOW

First make a list of some of your favorable qualities or virtues as a therapist—the things that you like about yourself and feel contribute to your effectiveness.

1.
2.
3.
4.
5.

Now look at each item on the list above and describe its opposite below on the corresponding numbered line:

1.
2.
3.
4.
5.

Picture a person who embodies these negative qualities. This is a rough portrait of your professional shadow.

Another interesting way to explore our professional shadow is to reflect on things you've done in your life, whether recently or in the more distant past, that you wouldn't want your patients to see. Why not?

Mindfulness practices facilitate the integration of our shadows by increasing awareness and acceptance. As we practice noticing what the mind is doing in each moment, we become more aware and accepting of all its elements, including those we don't like. Self-judgment becomes just another thought arising and passing in awareness. To the extent that we can accept our own imperfections in this way, our patients feel genuine trust and acceptance from us.

NOT KNOWING

There is a near-universal therapist secret that we rarely admit to our patients: Most of the time we don't know what we're doing. Early in our training we may have known. We may have taken courses that presented a theoretical model, met with supervisors who believed in that model, and interpreted our patients' difficulties accordingly. But once we have more experience, we discover we don't know as much as we thought we did (research suggests that clinicians generally become more flexible in orientation as they grow in professional experience [Auerbach & Johnson, 1977; Schacht, 1991]).

Let's say a patient presents with depression. Might it be anger turned against the self, perhaps because he or she wasn't able to express aggression toward caregivers (Freud's [1917] view)? Or might it be learned helplessness, based on repeated disappointments (Seligman's [1975] view)? Or is it an ecopsychological problem: The patient is alienated from community, family, and work living in an urban, industrialized culture? Or is the patient simply suffering from a serotonin imbalance for which an SSRI is the answer?

Knowing we don't know is helpful for establishing therapeutic alliances. Without this knowledge, we become like the mythical Greek figure Procrustes. He lived in a fortress near a major thoroughfare and would regularly invite passing travelers to spend the night. In his fortress he had a grand iron bed. If the traveler was too long for the bed, no problem—he'd cut off his feet. If the traveler was too short, he'd stretch him out to fit.

This is what our minds do when we are attached to a theory or hypothesis about a patient's distress. We tend to ignore or modify any information that doesn't fit that theory and elaborate that which supports it. In Piaget's (1952) terms, we readily *assimilate* information into our existing schemas, but find it difficult to *accommodate* our models to new data.

In our quest to be helpful or feel competent, it is easy to adopt simplistic, reductionistic understandings of our patients' difficulties. "It's because of his narcissistic mother," "It's a reaction to childhood neglect," "She's a borderline," and countless other conclusions help us to feel more secure as therapists, while overlooking our patients' complexity.

Mindfulness practices can help us avoid this trap. By practicing open monitoring during the session (see Chapters 1 and 5), we can see our thoughts and interpretations arising and passing, and consequently can learn to hold them more lightly. Initially it can be quite frightening to let go of our moorings in this way. It feels a bit like jumping out of an airplane without a parachute—a terrifying experience—until we realize that there is no ground (Fulton, 2013). We don't actually go *splat*; rather, we simply open to the next experience, idea, or understanding. Practicing mindfulness in this way allows us to develop what the Zen master Shunryu Suzuki (1973) called *beginner's mind*—the ability to let go of prior conceptions and see things with fresh eyes. As he famously put it, "In the beginner's mind there are many possibilities, but in the expert's there are few" (p. 21).

You can try this beginner's mind practice during a psychotherapy session.

BEGINNER'S MIND

- Before a therapy session, reflect for a few moments on the assumptions you hold about the nature of your patient's difficulties. What is causing his or her suffering? What might be the path through this?

- Settle into your seat at the beginning of the session. Become aware of the body, breath, and the experience of being present with your patient.

- As your patient speaks, note what thoughts arise in your mind. Notice each time your patient does or says something that confirms your assumptions about him or her, and how your mind reacts to these moments.

- Notice also anything that your patient does or says that doesn't fit your assumptions. See how the mind and heart react to these moments.

- As the session unfolds, notice any attachment you have to thinking you know what's happening and what you should do. Try deliberately to open to the uncertainty of the moment.

- After the session ends, take a moment to reflect on whether your view of your patient's difficulties have changed.

W.A.I.T.

As we realize that we often don't know what we're doing as therapists, we also realize that it might therefore be skillful to practice restraint. One of the fruits of learning to sit with uncomfortable feelings is the possibility of opening a gap between impulse and action. By sitting with bodily and emotional discomfort in meditation practice, we learn that we can feel a desire arise and have a choice whether to act on it. At more advanced stages of mindfulness practice, we become aware of the sequence that precedes behavior: a sensation arises, immediately accompanied by a feeling tone (like it, don't like it), followed by an intention (want it to continue, want it to end) and then action (doing something to hold on to a pleasant experience or end an unpleasant one).

In therapy, often the action at the end of this sequence is talking. While animated spontaneity can be a valuable therapist quality that enlivens the therapeutic relationship, impulsivity and compulsivity can get in the way. Many empathic failures occur when we act first and think later. As the old psychoanalytic maxim puts it, "The right interpretation at the wrong time is the wrong interpretation."

If we're attentive to the sequence by which an impulse turns into action, we may realize that sometimes we talk to forward the therapeutic enterprise, but other times our words are actually designed to help us feel that we're making a meaningful contribution, to interrupt a silence that makes us uncomfortable, or even to pursue the pleasure of telling a good story.

A simple way to make wiser decisions about speaking is to remind ourselves regularly of the acronym W.A.I.T.: <u>W</u>hy <u>A</u>m <u>I</u> <u>T</u>alking? Reflecting on this simple question will often illuminate what we're feeling at the moment and what our motivation is for speaking. Being mindful of this question can help keep therapy on track, and in so doing enhance our therapeutic alliance.

RELATIONAL MINDFULNESS

Despite having been refined by monks, nuns, and hermits, whose interpersonal relationships are constrained by detailed rules, mindfulness practices can help us navigate the complex nuances of more chaotic interpersonal relationships—including therapy relationships. Chapter 2 mentions that mindfulness practices can contribute to interpersonal attunement. Since many practices are solitary, this relational process often begins with developing *intra*personal attunement (Bruce, Manber, Shapiro, & Constantino, 2010). As we practice attending to the ever-changing kaleidoscope of inner experience, we become more aware of the thoughts, feelings, sensations, and reactions unfolding in our minds and bodies. This heightened awareness forms a foundation for *inter*personal attunement, which seems to rely on the mirror neuron system (Carr, Iacaboni, Dubeau, Mazziotta, & Lenzi, 2003; Iacaboni, 2009) to sense the mental state of another. We need intrapersonal attunement to be able to feel the activity of this system. As Carl Rogers (1961) famously said, empathy is the ability "to sense the client's private world as if it were your own, but without ever losing the 'as if' quality" (p. 284). Rogers's definition includes another contribution of mindfulness practice that we've been discussing—the ability to maintain perspective, tolerate discomfort, and not become completely identified with our emotional experience.

Three Objects of Awareness

Janet Surrey (2005) has suggested a way that therapists can approach each session as a mindfulness practice designed to enhance interpersonal attunement. It involves mindfully attending to three objects of awareness: (1) the sensations, thoughts, and feelings arising in "me"; (2) the words, body language, and sensed feeling experience of the patient; and (3) the flow of relationship, our felt sense of connection or distance. This last object of awareness can be the most elusive at first, but by developing the intention to notice it, we can become more adept at sensing when we are more or less connected with our patient.

THREE OBJECTS OF AWARENESS

- Settle into your seat at the beginning of the session. Become aware of your body, breath, and feeling state. Notice what thoughts and emotions are present.

- Now bring your attention to the words, body language, and facial expressions of your patient. See if you can sense in your own body his or her felt experience.

- Next notice your felt sense of connection or disconnection. Do you feel close to your patient at this moment? Does your patient seem to feel connected with you?

- As the session unfolds, continue to bring your attention to these three objects of awareness. Notice how they each change from moment to moment.

- As the session draws to a close and you consider your next meeting, notice your sense of connection or disconnection with your patient.

Life in a Space Suit

We all suffer from broken hearts. Loving other people involves countless injuries. From early moments in which our caregivers were inattentive, to feeling unwanted on the playground or rejected by a boyfriend or girlfriend, even those of us who have lived charmed lives have suffered deeply. Naturally, we erect all sorts of defenses to keep our hearts from breaking again. We may objectify others, labeling and categorizing them to avoid fully feeling our shared humanity. We may keep our more tender feelings to ourselves, taking care not to let others know how much they matter to us. Or we may simply turn our attention away from other people, becoming involved in safer pursuits.

All of these maneuvers separate us from one another. Ironically, while we imagine that they will keep us safe, they ultimately leave us more vulnerable. For when misfortune strikes and we're in pain, we're left to struggle with it alone, without the comfort of loving connection.

There is a legend of a lost paradise called Shambhala that predated the arrival of Buddhism in Tibet. In this kingdom, the highest attainment was to become a Shambhala warrior (Trungpa, 1988). These were not warriors in the conventional sense—they didn't have swords or spears. Instead, they were psychological warriors. It is said that they had the courage to live life *like a cow without its skin*, completely and exquisitely sensitive to all of their feelings.

While, as mentioned in Chapter 1, mindfulness practices can be used defensively to reinforce our isolation, they also have the potential to reduce it. They do this in part by helping us to be Shambhala warriors. As we've been discussing, mindfulness practice builds affect tolerance by teaching us that we can stay with painful experience and by showing us the impersonal nature of emotions. If we use this practice to enter into relationships deliberately, with the intention to accept whatever feelings arise, it can help connect us to others.

The following exercise requires a willing partner, ideally someone with some meditation experience. It can be a bit intense, but can enliven our relationships, help us appreciate our shared humanity, and bring us into connection with each other (allow about 30 minutes; adapted from R. D. Siegel, 2010).

BREATHING TOGETHER

- Begin by sitting facing each other, spines relatively erect. Close your eyes, and bring your attention to the sensations of your breath in your belly. Notice how your belly rises with each inhalation and falls with each exhalation. Whenever you find your attention wandering, gently return it to the sensations of the breath. You may notice some feelings of anxiety or apprehension doing this while facing another person. Just allow those feelings to come and go, returning your attention to the breath. Continue for 10 to 15 minutes.

- Once you've developed a little bit of concentration, gently open your eyes. Allow your gazes to rest on each other's bellies. Watch the breath of your partner as you also continue to notice the rising and falling sensations in your own body. Perhaps your breathing will start to synchronize; perhaps it won't. Either way, just try to remain aware of your own breathing and that of your partner for the next 5 minutes.

- The next phase can feel rather intense, so feel free to adjust your gaze as you see fit. Try raising your gaze to silently look into the eyes of your partner. Don't try to communicate anything in particular—just take in the experience of being with him or her.

- Allow yourself to notice your breath in the background while you focus most of your attention on looking into your partner's eyes. If this starts to feel too uncomfortable, feel free to lower your gaze to your partner's belly again, or even to close your eyes. You can shift back and forth between the belly and the eyes to adjust the intensity of this experience.

- Once you've gazed into your partner's eyes for several minutes, begin to imagine what he or she was like as a young child. Imagine him or her having a mother and father and growing up with other children. Imagine how he or she went through the same stages you did—going off to school, becoming a teenager, perhaps eventually leaving home. Be aware that your partner has had thousands of moments of joy and sorrow, fear and anger, longing and fulfillment—just like you. Go through the stages of life slowly, one by one.

- Now begin to imagine how your partner will look as he or she gets older. Be aware that, just like you, your partner will be dealing with the next stages of the life cycle. He or she will probably have to wrestle with infirmity and old age. Imagine how this will be for him or her—both the pleasant and unpleasant aspects.

- Finally, be aware that, just like you, someday your partner will die. The molecules in his or her body will recycle back into the earth or atmosphere and be transformed into something else.

- Once you've imagined your partner at all stages of the life cycle, bring your attention back to how he or she looks in the

present. Then drop your gaze down to your partner's belly
and breathe together again for a few minutes.

• Finish the exercise with several minutes of meditation
with your eyes closed. Notice the different feelings that
accompany each phase of the exercise.

• Finally, open your eyes, and take some time to discuss the
experience with your partner.

Available in audio at *www.sittingtogether.com*.

This exercise, along with several others presented in Chapter 6,
can help us to develop compassion for ourselves and our patients. This
compassion becomes grounded in a genuine appreciation of our shared
humanity, the fact that life is difficult for us all, as illness, decay, countless
disappointments, and death are part of everyone's reality. Our patients
can sense when we're not seeing them as "other," but recognize them
as fellow travelers, fellow suffering beings. This feeling of recognition
can be healing, as it allows patients to feel part of the human family, a
powerful antidote to the lonely isolation of most psychological distress.

TRANSITIONING TO MINDFULNESS-BASED TREATMENT

The next chapters introduce exercises that we can use to deepen our
own mindfulness practice, and that we can also teach to our patients.
Clinicians are often concerned that introducing these practices might
disrupt therapeutic alliances—especially if until now they had not
introduced structured exercises into treatment. By following a few
guidelines, we can minimize this possibility.

As discussed in Chapter 1, it's important to keep in mind your
patient's cultural background and identifications. Some patients will
find it much easier to try these practices if they're presented in a purely
secular framework, perhaps bolstered by research data, while others
will find it easier, and more meaningful, to engage with practices
presented from a religious or spiritual perspective. Explicitly asking
patients about their cultural backgrounds and religious or philosophic
beliefs can help you decide which approach to take.

Once deciding to introduce a particular practice, it's usually best
to present it as an experiment, suggesting that many people in similar
circumstances have found it to be useful. Here we tread a fine line

between encouraging positive expectations and motivating our patient to practice, versus risking setting him or her up for disappointment if the effect of the practice isn't as desired. If it fits with the nature of the therapeutic relationship, it can be useful to share your personal experience with the practice as one example of the effects it might have, as well as to share information gathered from research studies. For some patients, describing the expected neurobiological effects of practice can be motivating, especially since the hoped for effects may not be immediately apparent.

If you've been engaged in treatment with a patient for some time and have not introduced exercises previously, a bit of explanation is usually helpful. You may offer an honest description of your own exposure to the practice, or perhaps a discussion of your patient's current difficulties or developmental status and why mindfulness practice may be suited to his or her needs. Most patients have little difficulty shifting gears as long as the therapist is comfortable making the shift and offers a reasonable explanation for it.

It's best to introduce most practices early during a therapy session so that you can monitor their effects, make adjustments as necessary, and have time to help your patient integrate the experience. After about 5 minutes of practice, you might suggest, "Now stay with . . . [the breath or other object of awareness], and give me a status report. What are you noticing?" Most patients will be able to provide feedback without markedly interrupting the practice experience. It can be very useful to hear, for example, "I don't understand it, but I keep getting a creepy image of my father standing at my bedroom door when I was a little girl," or "This isn't working—I can't get my thoughts to stop," or "I'm very uncomfortable—I feel like I can't breathe." Receiving this feedback will allow you to modify or perhaps gently reiterate instructions to allow your patient to practice more easily.

It is usually helpful to elicit this sort of feedback at several points during the practice session, as well as to discuss the experience afterward. It's also usually encouraging for the therapist to engage in the practice along with the patient, even as the therapist provides ongoing instruction.

If, after adjusting the practice instructions, your patient is still uncomfortable with a particular practice, it's usually best to set it aside. This can be done in a normalizing way, explaining that different people respond differently to different practices, and you're happy to try another approach.

If, on the other hand, your patient seems to engage well with the practice, assigning additional practice as homework will probably be helpful. Recording meditation instructions based on the scripts found throughout this book in your own voice, and giving them to your patient to use, can add the support of the therapeutic alliance to your patient's meditation practice. Alternately, you can direct patients to the online reproducible handouts and audio recordings of selected practices that are available without charge at *www.sittingtogether.com*. Later, in Chapter 8, we explore how to introduce mindfulness practices to patients who may be particularly reluctant to try them. Then, in Chapter 9, we present illustrations of how various practices can be introduced and sequenced throughout the course of treatment. Additional varieties of meditation practice suited to the needs of particular individuals, along with further tips about which practices to use when, can also be found in the Appendix.

But first let's look more carefully at the core skills that comprise mindfulness, and the various practices that we and our patients can use to cultivate them.

CHAPTER FOUR

Concentration Practice

Focusing the Mind

Meditation is not an escape from life . . . but preparation
for really being in life.
—THICH NHAT HANH (in Murphy, 2002, p. 84)

Concentration, or focused attention, is the foundation of
meditation, the building block on which we base our practice. Jon
Kabat-Zinn (1994) calls it the "cornerstone" of mindfulness. Other
meditation practices, such as open monitoring, loving-kindness, and
compassion depend on this skill, which can be an anchor to which we
can return whenever we become distracted or overwhelmed.

What is concentration? Simply put, it is learning to steady and
calm our minds in the present moment. It is not an esoteric skill but
one that we use regularly in our daily lives. We employ concentration
in virtually everything we do, whether playing baseball, driving a car,
learning an instrument, or practicing yoga.

Because we juggle so many things, however, we are often stressed,
distracted, or only partially present. We half-listen to our children

telling us about their days while we cook dinner and check our phone for messages from suicidal patients. The nonstop demands of ordinary life often leave us scattered and exhausted. Concentration helps us reclaim our energy, to be rejuvenated. Instead of multitasking to keep up, adding more and more things to our to-do list, concentration helps us slow down and rest.

Concentration can be cultivated by paying attention to sounds, to the body, to the breath, and in some forms of meditation, to a phrase or a word. The practice is simple, but not necessarily easy. It involves bringing attention back to an object of awareness, without judgment or criticism, each time the mind wanders. It's like training a puppy. Just as we wouldn't beat or berate the puppy, we learn not to be harsh with ourselves when the mind wanders. It is simply its nature. We don't start calling ourselves "stupid" or "a bad meditator." We learn that it is OK to begin again, even after our mind has wandered thousands of times. As meditation teacher Jack Kornfield (1993) puts it, "In learning concentration, we feel as if we are always starting over, always losing our focus" (p. 62). We learn to befriend ourselves in the process. Kornfield adds, "Always remember that in training a puppy we want to end up with the puppy as our friend. In the same way, we practice seeing our mind and body as 'friend.'"

Though this practice may appear to be simple, it has profound implications. We learn to let go of ruminations about the past, not dwell on our mistakes or regrets, and not spin out so readily into fantasies and dreams about the future. We come back to what is actually happening in the present moment—the sounds around us, the feeling of our body sitting, the sensations of our breath. Like most worthwhile endeavors, this takes practice.

In concentration practice we don't try to suppress thoughts or feelings, as this only strengthens their hold. Instead, we note what has captured our attention and then gently return to the object of concentration, without self-loathing or judgment. In fact, this moment of realization that the mind has wandered is very valuable. As Sharon Salzberg (1997) suggests, instead of being an obstacle, this chance to begin again is the very "essence" of meditation.

> We may be lost in the past, lost in the future, or lost in judgment, but once we realize that we have been distracted, right in that moment we can begin again. . . . As we practice in this

way—seeing that no matter what outrageous, difficult, seductive, or foolish thought has arisen, we can begin again—a deep trust in ourselves takes shape. (p. 29)

Concentration practice also builds emotional resilience. Meditation teacher Christina Feldman (1998) points out that through the development of concentration the mind becomes "less fragile and susceptible to extremes. It becomes steady and balanced—able to receive the variety of experiences and impressions that come to us in life without feeling overwhelmed or burdened" (p. 23).

PAYING ATTENTION TO POSTURE

Meditation can be done sitting, standing, walking, or lying down. When sitting, there is no need to turn one's body into a pretzel by trying to get into a full lotus cross-legged position on a cushion. It is fine to sit comfortably on a chair, back upright, feet touching the floor. Hands can be resting in the lap or by the side. The body should be relaxed but alert, not stiff or rigid, not slumped or slouched. The eyes can be slightly open, softly focused on a spot on the floor a few feet away, or gently closed. With patients who are just starting, especially those who are anxious or have a trauma history, it is best to keep the eyes open.

Many of us have two primary modes of being: tense, goal-oriented activity or unfocused, often sleepy relaxation. Meditation cultivates a third mode of being simultaneously alert, awake, and relaxed. When practicing sitting meditation, assuming an alert, dignified physical posture can support this. Meditation teachers therefore often suggest sitting in a way that embodies one's essential dignity, an instruction that most people intuitively understand and find deeply affirming.

MAKING CONCENTRATION PRACTICE ACCESSIBLE TO PATIENTS

While meditation classes often begin with meditation on the breath, for many patients, particularly those with anxiety, trauma, or respiratory illness, this is not the best way to start. For these patients, as well as those who may be skeptical, the practice of listening to sounds is generally safer and more accessible.

SIMPLY LISTENING

- Start by sitting comfortably, eyes either slightly open or gently closed.
- Allow yourself to simply listen to the sounds around you. Notice the sounds of the traffic, the wind, the rain, the birds, or the air conditioner.
- There is no need to name the sounds, to grasp or hold on to them, or to push them away. Just allow yourself to listen to the sounds as they are.
- Imagine that your body is a gigantic ear or, if you prefer, a satellite dish, picking up 360 degrees of sound—above, below, in front, behind—all around you. Listen with your entire being.
- Notice that each sound has a beginning, middle, and end.
- If your mind wanders, no problem. Just bring it back to the present moment.
- Let yourself rest in the sounds of the moment, knowing that this moment is unique and that this constellation of sounds will never be repeated.
- Take a deep breath, wiggle your fingers and toes, stretch, and open your eyes if they have been closed. Try to extend focused attention into your next activity.

Available in audio at *www.sittingtogether.com*.

Sharon Salzberg and Joseph Goldstein (2001) explain the benefits of beginning with sound:

> We begin with hearing because it points to something of the natural quality of mindfulness. We don't have to make the sounds come or go. We don't have to identify them; we don't have to manipulate them. We can hear sounds without having to make any effort to do so. The object of sound appears, and we're present . . . we're alert . . . we connect to it." (p. 32)

CLINICAL ILLUSTRATION: ONE SOUND AT A TIME

Margaret came to treatment to help deal with her stress. She was trying to balance a full-time job and three children. Her mother had recently had a stroke, and Margaret was managing her medical care in addition to carpooling, running the house, taking the kids to soccer practice, and meeting the demands of her job. Feeling overwhelmed, she consulted her primary care physician who suggested she try meditation.

Margaret was skeptical about mindfulness practice but thought it was worth a try since she didn't want to take "yet another pill." When she started, she experienced her mind racing, dancing from one responsibility to the next. She complained that it didn't seem to be working and wondered if meditation was really appropriate for someone with such a busy life. Her therapist responded by explaining that many people feel this way, and the practice really is a lot like puppy training, required a lot of patience and self-acceptance. Desperate to feel less stressed, she tried brief daily practice sessions and eventually found she could return to the present moment, "one sound at a time." It was hard to find time in her schedule, but she managed to set aside 5 minutes a day and practice informally in the midst of her other tasks. She reported a greater sense of ease and even felt her sense of humor return as she shuttled between her mother's rehab and her son's soccer games, tuning in to the sounds around her whenever she became stressed or agitated. "I feel like I've discovered a new addition to my house," she joked, "there is all this extra space in my mind."

Sharon Salzberg (1997) details a variety of different responses to listening meditation that can be useful to present to patients:

> There are so many ways to hear a sound. We might hear a certain noise and become reactive and upset, finding it unpleasant. If we think the sound is a pleasant one, we might want it to go on and on. If the sound strikes us as neither pleasant nor unpleasant, however, we may only "half-hear" it. Or, we can hear a sound directly, without judgment or conceptual elaboration—simply as a sensory event—and the whole world can open up before us. (pp. 39–40)

Composer John Cage, a student of Zen Buddhism, became famous for what he called his "melodies of silence." In his most famous and controversial composition, *4'33"*, the performer sits at a piano without ever touching the keys. The "music" that the audience hears are the natural sounds in the room (Murphy, 2002). Adapting Cage's experiment, we can engage patients and introduce listening practice by suggesting that we are listening to a symphony performed solely for us in this moment.

Connecting with the Body

This next practice, *Touch Points*, is another excellent tool to develop concentration. In this meditation, the patient is instructed to bring attention to the places where the body is "touching"—such as the eyes, lips, hands, legs, and feet. It is a way to ground awareness in the body, which in turn helps calm the mind. Because the attention is on the periphery of the body, this is usually a good practice for those with a history of trauma or emotional deregulation who need to establish safety.

TOUCH POINTS

- Start by sitting comfortably, assuming a posture of dignity with your spine erect and your feet touching the ground. Eyes can be slightly open with a soft gaze or gently closed.
- Take three or four breaths to let the mind and body settle and come into the present moment.
- Notice the places where your body is "touching"—the eyelids touching, the lips touching, the hands touching, the sitting bones touching, the backs of the knees touching the chair, and the feet touching the ground.
- Repeat the sequence, finding a comfortable rhythm— attending to eyes touching, lips touching, hands touching, sitting bones touching, knees touching, feet touching. Note these touch points silently to yourself if it helps you focus.
- If you get distracted, no problem, no blame—just start again.
- When you are ready, take a deep breath, stretch, wiggle your fingers and toes, rotate your wrists and ankles, and open your eyes if they have been closed. Try to extend focused attention into your next activity.

Available in audio at *www.sittingtogether.com*.

CLINICAL ILLUSTRATION: NOT FEEDING THE ANGER

Richard entered treatment to work on anger. He found himself losing his temper with colleagues at work and with his wife and young children at home. Afraid he might lose his job or even hurt someone, his family insisted that he get help. Not surprisingly, Richard wasn't happy with this suggestion. But he had grown up with a physically violent and verbally abusive father and, humiliating as it was to enter treatment for anger difficulties, he didn't want his children, family, or colleagues to experience a similar terror.

Richard needed a lot of support around his anger before he was open to trying meditation. His therapist explored with him how natural it was, given his childhood, that he'd experience rage and then have difficulty restraining himself from expressing it. Once he felt understood and not pathologized, he was willing to try practicing with the touch points first in therapy and then at work and home. Occasionally, when a coworker made a mistake, instead of blowing up he learned to pause and bring his focus to the touch points. Sometimes he would have to repeat the sequence over and over, but it gave him an anchor for his attention that helped him contain his rage. At home, he started to practice at dinner, where he had been most volatile. If one of his children spilled something or talked back, Richard would return to his body, staying with the soles of his feet so as not to fly into a rage. It didn't always work, and he continued to struggle with shame about his anger, but he was grateful when he was able to restrain himself.

This practice has many clinical applications. Bringing attention to the soles of the feet helped a volatile, mentally disabled young man control his aggression (Singh, Wahler, Adkins, & Myers, 2003), and it is often used in anger management programs. This is also a useful technique for children who have trouble sitting still or paying attention. (See the Appendix.)

A variation on this practice is meditation on the hands, which is taught by Tara Brach (2003, 2011), as well as Williams, Teasdale, Segal, and Kabat-Zinn (2007). It is a concentration technique that we have found particularly effective with anxiety and some forms of obsessive–compulsive disorder (OCD), such as hand washing (see Pollak, 2013, for a clinical application).

While this practice is commonly done in the sitting posture, it can also be done lying down, where it is helpful in the treatment of insomnia.

CLINICAL ILLUSTRATION: SURRENDERING TO SLEEPLESSNESS

Juanita had a terrible time sleeping. She had a very stressful job in high tech and her firm had experienced massive layoffs. She felt she was doing the work of two or three people. Recently divorced, she also had been feeling the loneliness of the "empty nest" since her children had left for college. When she woke at two or three in the morning, she began to ruminate about the demise of her marriage and to worry that she would be alone for the rest of her life. This would spiral into concerns about growing old and facing illness and death without support. She woke up exhausted most mornings and often felt so foggy that her performance at work suffered.

Eager for any help she could get with her insomnia, Juanita experimented with a variation of the touch points practice when she couldn't sleep. She would notice her hands touching, her shoulders touching, her hips touching, her legs touching, and her feet touching. As she practiced, she noticed feelings of desperation about getting to sleep. With repeated practice, however, she learned to relax this pressure and stop fighting sleeplessness. The practice calmed and steadied her, and she learned to stay with the sensations of the present moment, not to project into an imaginary future or agonize about mistakes in the past.

Even though she didn't always fall back asleep, she felt more rested. With continued meditation she got less caught in ruminative loops. After 2 months of daily practice, sleep usually came more easily. On the nights that it didn't, Juanita still got upset, and feared she'd be exhausted the next day. But she also used these additional waking hours to meditate for a longer time. Her relationship with her negative thoughts began to shift and she reported that increasingly she could notice the thoughts, let them go, and then return to the touch points.

As Joseph Goldstein (1993) explains, when we cultivate concentration, whatever is happening in the mind is not as important as how we respond to it: "The key question is, how do we relate to what is arising? Are we relating to these emotions by thinking about them or analyzing them? Or are we relating by simply feeling and observing?" (p. 100). Instead of responding to her sleeplessness with agitation and worry, wondering how she would function the next day, Juanita learned to *be with* her experience. The goal became not to get rid of fear and anxiety but to learn more skillful ways to be with it.

Working with the Breath

The practice of focusing attention on the breath is a core concentration practice. The breath is always available as an object of awareness. The practice has been successfully used for over 2,500 years, and is portable and nondenominational—no particular belief system is required to employ it.

For patients who are relatively well integrated, concentrating attention on the breath is an excellent practice. For those who are dissociative, have a trauma history, or struggle with intense anxiety, it is usually better to work with the practices of *Listening, Touch Points*, or *Walking Meditation* (see Chapter 5). In breath practice we attend to the natural breath without forcing or manipulating it. We learn to settle into the breath and the awareness of the present moment. We let go of judgments and criticisms, allowing the breath to be as it is—constantly moving and always changing. Like all meditation practices, working with the breath requires a willingness to repeatedly begin again. When we get overwhelmed, lost in the past, captured by thought, anger, or regret, we can always reconnect with the breath. Meditation teacher Larry Rosenberg (2004) says, if you "have to come back a thousand times in a five minute period of sitting, just do it. It's not a problem unless you make it into one" (p. 34). Since most people are alarmed to discover just how unruly their mind is, it's helpful to repeatedly emphasize that having our attention hijacked by thoughts and feelings is normal for beginning and experienced meditators alike.

FINDING THE BREATH

- Start by sitting comfortably, assuming a posture of dignity with your back straight, your spine relaxed but not rigid, eyes either softly open or closed.
- Find your breath. We are often so busy that we often don't realize that we are breathing. Simply notice your breath.
- See where you feel your breath most strongly. It may be at the nostrils, at the chest, or in the belly. Allow yourself to feel the sensations of each inhalation and exhalation.
- If your mind wanders, no problem. Give yourself permission to begin again.
- Gently, kindly bring yourself back. Let the breath become your anchor, your friend. Rest in your breath.
- Don't be too ambitious; take it slow. We all have the ability to feel one breath completely.
- When you are ready, stretch, wiggle fingers and toes, and open the eyes if they have been closed. Try to extend focused attention into your next activity.

Available in audio at *www.sittingtogether.com*.

Bonnie, a woman in her 20s, lost her job in an economic downturn. She became depressed, feeling she was a failure. Her parents kept nagging her to look for work, which only made things worse. Discouraged about her job prospects, she spent more and more time playing computer games.

Bonnie did not want to take medication but was willing to try meditation. She was generally high functioning and well integrated. As she began to practice, she found the permission to begin again was a huge relief, something that had been absent in her upbringing. She began to realize that it was not a moral failing to be out of work, her joblessness need not define her, and she probably would not be unemployed forever. As she relaxed and noticed how her breath was not static but constantly changing and moving, she became less fearful of other change in her life. She learned to embrace the fluidity rather than retreat into computer games. The breath became both metaphor and motivation. By learning to "begin again" in her practice of meditation, she realized that it was OK to begin again in her life as well. As she noticed the suffering she was creating by blaming herself, she realized that she was making a difficult situation even worse. Reflecting on what it meant to "start again" without judgment, condemnation, or criticism, she reconnected with a career aspiration that her parents had dismissed as "impractical," giving herself permission to take a risk and try something new.

Bonnie's father had held one job for his entire life, so she had no model for starting over. Not only were such jobs rare these days, she actually didn't *want* a job for life. She wanted to explore and try new things. Starting again gives people permission to break habitual patterns. As Sharon Salzberg (2011) puts it:

> The moment you realize you've been distracted is the magic moment. It's a chance to be really different, to try a new response—rather than tell yourself you're weak or undisciplined, or give up in frustration, simply let go and begin again. In fact, instead of chastising yourself, you might thank yourself for recognizing that you've been distracted, and for returning to your breath. (p. 49)

At times, when the mind is agitated and following the breath is difficult, it can be helpful to give the mind something additional on which to focus. Meditation teachers suggest silently noting "rising" during an inhalation and "falling" during an exhalation, or noting "in" and "out" as the breath enters and leaves the body. Many people also find that counting is a helpful aid to concentration. Noting "one" with the inhalation and "two" with the exhalation is also an excellent practice, as is creating a game, counting breaths to 10 but beginning again whenever we lose track of the breath. Feel free to experiment. The important thing to remember, as the Thai meditation master Ajahn Chah says, "is to keep it simple and stay in the present moment" (Rosenberg, 2004, p. 26).

CLINICAL ILLUSTRATION: DOING IT BY THE NUMBERS

John was a middle-aged man who worked as an accountant. He entered treatment to deal with social anxiety. He had tried a meditation class at his local YMCA but found it "boring" and had trouble focusing his attention. While he felt that he was a "failure" at meditation, after reading that it could change the brain, he wanted to give it another chance. He experimented with a few different methods and found that silently counting was a good fit—he lived in a world of numbers and felt comfortable incorporating them in his meditation.

John began to experiment with bringing mindfulness more fully into his life. He noticed his breath in anxious situations, such as during meetings at work or on dates. Staying with his breath, one breath at a time, he found that he could bear the discomfort of anxiety, knowing that it would pass and that he could always start again with the next breath. As he learned to stay in the moment, he found he was less focused on what he needed to say or do, which allowed him to listen to others more readily. This in turn improved his work and social relationships.

Many people worry that they can't meditate, that they're doing it "wrong." It can be helpful to point out to patients that they are already doing fine just by breathing, and that there is no way to fail at this practice—sitting down for even 2 minutes has benefits.

Many patients find that when they get in touch with the breath they also become aware of other emotions they've been carrying. The following variation, taught by Sharon Salzberg (2011), has the benefit of being less inner focused than other breath practices. Consequently, it can serve as a bridge between the touch points and traditional breath meditations, and can be used effectively with people who struggle with intense emotions, such as those who have experienced severe trauma or grief. If the patient is willing and able to work with intense feelings, this variation establishes a sense of comfort and of being held or "cradled," while attending to the breath.

CRADLING THE BREATH

- Start by sitting comfortably, letting yourself feel grounded and anchored in your chair or cushion. Get in touch with your essential dignity.
- Start with three or four deep breaths.
- As you bring your attention to where you feel your breath most strongly—the nostrils, the chest, or the belly, lovingly cradle each breath.
- Imagine that you can touch each breath with kindness and tenderness, as if you were holding a bird or something else precious and delicate.
- If intense feelings arise, see if you can cradle these as well. No need to explore them or analyze them, but allow yourself to notice and touch the emotions, and then return to the breath.

CLINICAL ILLUSTRATION: TOUCHING THE SADNESS

Tara, a single woman in her 50s, entered treatment to process her grief over her mother's recent death. It had been a long and difficult illness and her mother had been in severe pain. Tara had taken a leave from work to care for her. However, she had not been present at the actual moment of death and because of this was wracked by guilt. She was hoping that meditation might help her find some peace.

As she tried to find her breath, she found instead an ocean of tears. This made her think that meditation might not be such a good idea. Her therapist explained that the heart and mind push feelings out of awareness when they're initially too difficult to bear, and these tend to come flooding back in when we relax our usual busyness. It's not really a problem unless we don't feel ready to reintegrate the feelings.

This made sense to Tara, and she said that now was as good a time as any to feel her grief more fully. So she practiced holding her sorrow in her hands, cradling and containing it, and then returning to her breath. At first she could only do this for a few moments and she worried that her sorrow would be endless and would engulf her. As she moved back and forth between sorrow and breath, she developed an increased appreciation of the preciousness of the breath and the preciousness of life. With time, she was left with an appreciation of her mother's life and a desire to live the rest of her own life as fully as possible.

As we begin to open to our experience, we open to pain as well. As Ajahn Chah remarked, "If you haven't cried a number of times, your meditation hasn't really begun" (Kornfield, 1993, p. 40).

One of the key components of meditation is allowing ourselves to experience all that is happening at the moment—the pleasant, the unpleasant, and the neutral—without being drawn into it. We don't deny or hide from painful or unpleasant feelings, we just learn not to get caught up in them. We learn not to berate ourselves for having disturbing or violent thoughts, but we don't pretend they're not there, either. Meditation teachers often help students troubled by thoughts by saying, "Why are you so upset about the thought that came up in your mind? Did you invite it?" (Salzberg, 2011, p. 66). By noticing the thoughts and then returning to the breath without self-hatred or condemnation, we begin to release ourselves from the sway of negative thoughts and emotions.

The following practice is a departure from traditional approaches to talk therapy, at least in psychodynamic and humanistic traditions. We are used to delving in and processing the details of what happened in the past. However, at times we get stuck in our histories and can't extricate ourselves, so that they cause us more suffering. This is a useful practice to help shift therapy from the narrative to the experiencing mode discussed in Chapter 1.

LETTING GO OF THE STORY

- Sit comfortably, eyes either partly open or closed. Come into a posture of dignity.

- Find your breath where you feel it most strongly—the nostrils, the chest, or the abdomen. No need to judge it or control it, just feel your natural breath.

- When your mind begins to wander, getting lost in a story or drama, simply say to yourself, "Not now, just the breath."

- Gently return to the breath, even if your mind gets pulled away hundreds of times. Remind yourself, "Just the breath, nothing else."

- Notice what is distracting you, make a mental note of it, and then say to yourself, "Let me be with this breath now, let me feel this breath."
- When you are ready, stretch, wiggle your fingers and toes, and open your eyes if they have been closed. See if you can notice whenever your mind gets lost in thought throughout the rest of the day.

CLINICAL ILLUSTRATION: COMING INTO THE PRESENT

Paula and Brian entered couple therapy after a turbulent time in their marriage. Paula had been involved in an affair, but had ended it and recommitted to the marriage. Brian did not want the marriage to end, but was haunted by disturbing thoughts of Paula in bed with another man. Although he wanted to start over and give the marriage another chance, he couldn't let go of his anger, hurt, and humiliation.

As he began to explore his feelings of betrayal, he realized that he was getting caught in an endless loop, continually replaying fantasies of Paula with the other man. The affair had ended over 2 years ago, but in his mind it was still happening. Their therapist sensed that Brian's repetitive thoughts were not helping him to integrate his feelings about the betrayal, but had instead simply become an obsession.

Brian was encouraged to return to his breath when he felt trapped in obsessive thoughts about the other man. Over months of work, he was able to voice his feelings of betrayal and anger, as well as hear Paula's genuine love and commitment to him. They both acknowledged the courage and hard work it had taken to forge a different and more honest relationship. Whenever he returned to obsessing about the past, Brian would remind himself to drop the story and return to the present. He would notice his breath and appreciate what he and Paula had right now. By repeatedly practicing beginning again in his meditation, he was able to give the marriage another chance.

Informal Concentration Practice

Most of the meditation exercises we've been discussing can also be used as informal practices during the course of daily life. For example, listening to sounds can be done upon waking in the morning, walking, sitting on a bus or subway, or when listening to a partner, parent, child, or patient. (See also *Listening to Another* in the Appendix, p. 204) Connecting with the touch points can be used during a difficult conversation (grounding with the soles of the feet, softening and unclenching the hands) or throughout the day (and night) when potentially overwhelming emotions arise. Awareness of the breath is totally portable since the breath is always with us. We can notice the breath at a red light or stop sign or when we experience "road rage." We can tune into the breath while having a cup of tea or coffee or during a pause before picking up the phone or answering e-mail. Some therapists like to set aside a minute or two to breathe between patients as a way of letting go of the past session and opening to the next one. Finally, we can practice letting go of the story whenever we're stuck in obsessional thoughts or anger.

Being Realistic

Patients usually need frequent reminders that it's OK if meditation doesn't always feel good. Feeling good is not the goal, and concentration often doesn't come easily. Like any other skill, such as playing the piano, dancing, or learning tai chi, it takes practice. An analogy with developing physical fitness can often help. Sometimes we go to the gym and feel like our workout is nearly effortless, at other times the same workout is a struggle. While one feels better, we value both, knowing that on the more difficult day we're increasing our fitness at least as much as on the easy day.

Meditation practice also isn't just for good times, but is most useful for what Jon Kabat-Zinn (1990) calls the "full catastrophe" of life. When things are difficult, meditating can be more challenging, but also may be particularly useful for shifting our perspective, allowing us to grow through challenging experiences. As the ancient African saying reminds us, "Smooth seas do not make for skillful sailors."

WHAT DOES CONCENTRATION LOOK AND FEEL LIKE?

So how do we know if we (and our patients) are developing the skill of concentration or focused attention? In mindfulness practice, we rely on concentration to bring stability of mind to the present moment in order to investigate and look deeply into the full range of what life presents. When we get overwhelmed, it can be very helpful to return to the grounding practices of awareness of sounds, touch points, and the breath. These practices become a particularly valuable anchor when repressed or otherwise disavowed material begins to surface. So if we want to help our patients develop this skill, how can we assess their learning?

Sharon Salzberg (2011) presents helpful touchstones for identifying when concentration is present. As adapted here, these are guidelines, not rigid criteria. And, as always, it is important to be aware of and responsive to individual differences.

1. There is some present-moment awareness. This does not mean that we are present in every moment (no one is) but we can stay with the breath (or sounds, or touch points) for a few seconds at a time, enough to experience what full attention feels like.
2. We notice when we get distracted and are able to begin again. Even experienced meditators get distracted. We want to develop the ability to notice that our mind has wandered, catch ourselves, gather our attention, and return to the practice.
3. We practice letting go of criticism and judgment. Again, we don't expect to let go of all judgments, but we can allow our meditation practice to unfold without harsh criticism. We don't beat ourselves up when our mind wanders, we don't call our-selves names, we catch ourselves before spinning off into future catastrophic predictions.
4. We become kinder to ourselves. Life is hard for everyone. There is so much that we can't control. Meditation becomes a refuge from endless self-loathing. Through our practice we learn to befriend ourselves and plant the seeds of self-compassion.
5. We become aware of a stable, calm center that is usually available. We get less "hooked" by ruminative and obsessive thoughts. We feel less exhausted and more alive. For many, increased calmness and stability bring an experience of new energy and self-reliance.

How do we assess if our patients have developed a capacity for concentration? Often simply asking a patient about these touchstones is helpful. Bear in mind that our capacity for concentration may vary from day to day. In times of stress or difficulty, it is often more chal-lenging to concentrate and focus the mind. During these times, it can be helpful to set aside an additional time to practice, even if it is for a brief period, or to try different practices. For example, many patients find counting meditation helps anchor the mind when particularly distracted or preoccupied, and practices such as *Letting Go of the Story* can be especially useful when trapped in obsessive thinking.

The factors listed above come and go depending on the circumstances in the moment. As touchstones, they can help us get our bearings, to notice when concentration is present in our journey through the ever-changing terrain of our minds.

CHAPTER FIVE

Open Monitoring

Expanding the Mind

> Mindfulness is the energy that sheds light on all things and
> all activities . . . bringing forth deep insight and awakening.
> —Thich Nhat Hanh (1974, pp. 25–26)

Once we are able to establish some stability of mind through concentration practice, we can begin to explore the practice of mindfulness per se or what researchers call open monitoring. Mindfulness helps us see our lives more clearly. Meditation teachers compare open monitoring with a powerful searchlight that can illuminate all things as they arise in awareness. Teacher Sharon Salzberg (2011) uses the analogy of entering a dusty attic room and turning on the light:

> In that light we see everything—the beautiful treasures we're grateful to have unearthed; the dusty, neglected corners that inspire us to say, "I'd better clean that up"; the unfortunate relics of the past that we thought we had gotten rid of long ago. We acknowledge them all, with an open, spacious, and loving awareness. (pp. 128–129)

Open monitoring is invaluable in clinical work as it helps both patient and therapist stay present with suffering in all its forms. No matter how difficult a situation is, no matter what its history or how long a symptom has persisted, open monitoring can help us find a skillful way to work with what is happening in our lives at this moment. As we begin to open our minds, we become more skilled at noticing our automatic, conditioned responses. We develop a more accurate perception of what is actually happening, rather than relying on the stories we tell ourselves. Open monitoring reveals how our reactions add to our experience, not only in meditation but in life. When we practice this mindfulness skill, our efforts are not directed toward achieving a different transcendent state of mind, but toward seeing the ways we get trapped by fear, anxiety, anger, and desire. In a calm and accepting way, we learn to observe the functioning of our minds and gain insight into our behavior. We don't run away from our problems and difficulties; we turn consciously toward them.

In concentration practice we learn that sounds, the breath, and other objects of awareness come and go. In open monitoring, we bring that same awareness to whatever spontaneously arises in the mind, including thoughts, emotions, and images. We train our attention to see these contents as clouds moving across the sky, transient events rather than ultimate truths. Jack Kornfield (1993) observes that no state of mind, feeling, or emotion lasts more than 15 to 30 seconds. When we're mindful, we let these mind states come and go rather than grasping on to them, exaggerating them, or creating dramas because of them. We notice all that is happening—sounds, smells, thoughts, feelings— without holding on to what is pleasant, avoiding what is unpleasant, or ignoring what is neutral.

To recognize that our thoughts are just thoughts, and that our thoughts are not absolute truths, is liberating. We can realize that the painful beliefs we have held for years—that we are unlovable, bad, lazy, incompetent, or unworthy—are not necessarily true. Learning to let go of negative thoughts can help us break vicious cycles of rumination. Those thoughts no longer cause us to spiral down into a depressed mood or rev up into an anxious one. We often try to think our way out of our moods, only to get stuck in painful negative feedback loops. Mindfulness instead allows us to get unstuck and back in touch with our bodies, our wisdom, and our aliveness.

The power of open monitoring is revealed through continued practice. As we free ourselves from conditioned thinking, we can see more clearly and understand more deeply, gaining insight into issues we previously were unable or unwilling to examine openly. Courage and confidence build from being able to work with any difficulty or problem that arises, freeing us to experience more joy, pleasure, and happiness.

DEVELOPING AWARENESS OF THE BODY

The novelist James Joyce (1914/1991) understood that we are often disconnected from our bodies, and hence from the present moment, when he wrote: "Mr. Duffy . . . lived at a little distance from his body" (p. 71). In contrast, turning our attention to the body is a good way to discover what is happening in the moment, for as Tara Brach (2012) reminds us, "The body lives in the present" (p. 80). Since the body is always available as an object of meditation, becoming interested and curious about physical sensations is one of the easiest ways to come into the present moment. This practice can help us see the difference between direct experience and what we add on. Because many patients may be restless or initially have trouble sitting still, walking meditation can be a good starting place to connect with the body. It can provide a nice transition from concentration practice to open monitoring, and is a practice that easily moves from the consulting room into everyday life.

Walking meditation brings awareness to an activity we usually perform as if we're on "automatic pilot." So often we hurry to get somewhere, thinking about what we'll do or say when we get there, ignoring the process of walking. In this meditation we bring our attention to the experience of moving through space. While walking meditation can be done as a concentration practice, focusing on a single sensation, it readily transitions into open monitoring, especially when done outside, where so many sensations vividly present themselves.

WALKING MEDITATION: ANCHORING IN THE BODY

- Stand comfortably with your eyes open, feet about hip distance apart, weight evenly divided between the feet. Arms can be at your sides, behind you, or in front of you— whatever feels most comfortable. Let yourself feel connected to the ground.
- Become aware of any sensations in the toes, soles, and heels.

Feel free to shift your weight between the feet to make these sensations clearer.

- Start walking slowly, remaining relaxed and alert. Feel your feet touching the ground. Silently note to yourself "touching, touching."
- Bring attention to each movement of walking—lifting, moving, placing.
- Notice what is happening around you but keep your focus on the sensation of walking.
- If you find you're able to attend with some continuity to the sensations in your feet and legs, let your awareness expand to take in the light, colors, sounds, and smells around you. Notice whatever predominates in your awareness. No control, no effort, no explicit focus.
- If you get overwhelmed, or if your attention gets hijacked by trains of thought—no problem, bring yourself back to the feeling of your feet touching the ground.
- When you are ready to stop, return to your breath, the feeling of your feet on the ground, and stretch.
- See if you can carry this awareness into your next activity.

Available in audio at *www.sittingtogether.com*.

CLINICAL ILLUSTRATION: BEFRIENDING THE BODY

Barbara was a 17-year-old in treatment at an outpatient clinic at a large city hospital. She had a dual diagnosis of major depression and alcohol addiction. Barbara had been abused as a child and was severely obese. At first she resisted meditation, saying that it was "dumb." But she was willing to give it a try when her therapist framed it as an experiment, since biology was her favorite subject and she liked lab experiments. Her therapist started with *Simply Listening*, and together they listed all the sounds they noticed (see Chapter 4, page 68). Barbara liked this exercise and found it soothing. Given her age and history, sitting still was not easy for her, so her therapist's next suggestion was walking meditation. Barbara took to it right away.

Barbara would enter the tiny, windowless office in the clinic, look around and with a smile say, "Let's blow this joint." Barbara and her therapist began by walking around the grounds of the hospital, at first just bringing attention to the sensation of the feet touching the ground.

They walked together like this for months, usually spending a few minutes in silence before beginning to talk.

Barbara had never felt comfortable in her body, so learning to bring kind attention to each step was a new experience. She had always thought of her body as an enemy and viewed it as a source of shame. As a result, she was constantly berating herself with negative thoughts: "Why are you so fat? You are such a lazy pig! Why can't you get your act together?" Gradually, Barbara felt empowered to take other steps. She started walking by herself, enjoying the quiet that was so different from the constant noise and fighting in her house. When she had a hard day, she especially enjoyed the variation of *Silly Walking* (see the Appendix, p. 208). She eventually joined a 12-step program, where she found additional support for dealing with her addictions, her overeating, and her trauma.

Some patients wonder if walking practice is really meditation. It is. While the outward form may not be what they expect, the intention is the same as in sitting practice. Meditation can be practiced sitting, standing, walking, and lying down. But with walking meditation, unlike regular walking, we are not trying to go anywhere. Instead, we are learning to be fully present with every step.

While it is nice to have a large, open space to walk, this isn't necessary. Walking can be done in a small office in a circle or back and forth. The point is to bring awareness to the sensations of movement in the present moment. It can also be useful to practice simply standing upright. This, along with walking practice, can be a nice alternative to sitting practice when we are sleepy. Children and adolescents also do well with variations of walking practice (see *Silly Walking* in the Appendix). For those with disabilities, walking can be modified in other ways. One patient focused on the hand movement of pushing her wheelchair, feeling the motion in her hands rather than in her feet.

The following practice is taught by Narayan Helen Liebenson at Cambridge Insight Meditation Center. Like walking practice, it tends to open our awareness to a wide range of sensations, inclining the mind toward open monitoring. It can be practiced sitting, standing, or lying down. Because it brings awareness to the periphery of the body, it is a relatively safe and nonthreatening way to focus attention on the body, and is therefore suitable for people with not fully integrated traumatic memories or those who have difficulty tolerating their emotions. Many patients find that they can use this meditation during breaks in the day both at work and at home, or when doing repetitive activities such as filing or washing dishes. This meditation brings awareness to both the front and back of the body, which is sometimes neglected in traditional meditation instructions.

BODY SWEEP

- Sit or stand comfortably. Take a few breaths to come into the present moment, realizing where you are now, not dwelling in the past or worrying about the future.

- Using your mind's eye, imagine that you can "sweep" down the area between the top of the head and eyes, bringing attention to the periphery of the body, noticing any tension or tightness in the forehead and inviting it to soften and relax. Then sweep the area from your eyes to your chin, noticing any sensations in the jaw, inviting the muscles to soften.

- Next sweep from the chin to the collarbone, letting the neck and throat soften. Pause to notice what is happening. Bring attention from the collarbone to the shoulders, noticing the sensations and, if you like, breathing into any tension or tightness. From the shoulders sweep through the chest, pausing, then sweep down to the stomach, pausing, breathing into any sensations or tightness. Notice what is present without judgment or criticism. Sweep down from the stomach to the hip bones, pausing and noticing any sensations.

- Return to the shoulders and sweep down both arms simultaneously, pausing at the elbows and wrists, then resting at the fingers. Just notice what sensations are present in the body.

- From the hips sweep down through the pelvis, pausing to feel any sensations, and then down the thighs, resting at the knees, with awareness and interest. From the knees sweep down through the ankles and out through the toes.

- Now bring attention to the parts of the body we usually don't notice. Sweep the soles of the feet, from the toes to the heels. Then proceed up the back of the body, sweeping from the heels to the knees, becoming aware of any sensations, any clenching or tightness. Allow the muscles to soften.

- Move from the backs of the knees to the buttocks, bringing kind attention to the sensations. Again, no judgment, no criticism. Move from the buttocks to the lower back, pausing to notice sensations in the back. Notice any discomfort that is held in the back, inviting it to soften. Sweep from the lower back to the mid-back to the shoulder blades, bringing awareness to sensations as well as any discomfort.

- From the shoulder blades sweep down the backs of both arms simultaneously, noticing in order the upper arms, the elbows, the wrists, and the palms.

- Return to the shoulders, sweeping up through the neck to the back of the head, pausing and noticing any sensations or discomfort.

- Finally, sweep up from the back of the head and ears, coming to rest at the crown of the head.

- In the last few minutes, allow your attention to go to whatever sensations are most vivid in each moment. Open your awareness to the world around you. Let sounds come to you. If your eyes have been closed, gently open them. Notice the light, shadows, and colors. Notice perhaps your feet touching the floor, the feel of your buttocks on the chair or cushion, any other sensations that arise. Let your mind be free, exerting no effort, no control.

- When you are ready, wiggle fingers and toes, and stretch. Try to remain mindful during your next activity.

CLINICAL ILLUSTRATION: INHABITING THE BODY

Amy worked as a hairdresser, which meant she spent most of the day on her feet. She had taken a new job in an upscale salon, where she felt intimidated. Her boss was critical, complaining that she talked too much and worked too slowly. After 3 stressful months, she was placed on probation.

Amy found herself not wanting to get out of bed or go to work. She had limited education, low self-esteem, and mild attention deficit disorder (ADD). Her mother had constantly criticized her, so it was especially difficult for her to stomach her boss's micromanagement. She began to feel nausea and panic every morning. Her finances were limited and she couldn't afford to lose this job.

Initially Amy had no interest in meditation, saying it wasn't for her and refusing to try it. "Can't I just take a fucking pill to make the anxiety go away? I want to talk, I don't like silence, it makes me nervous." Given the intensity of her resistance, her therapist did not push.

However, a number of months later, her best friend told her that meditation would help with job stress. Her friend was using an online meditation app and noticed a difference. Feeling desperate about losing her job, Amy said she was willing to try. She liked listening to sounds, but "hated" feeling the breath. "It makes me want to run outa here," she said. As the *Body Sweep* was something that she could do on the job, it seemed like a good next step. Amy liked it and began to practice it at work. When she noticed her boss watching her, she brought her attention to her body, sweeping down the front and up the back to center herself. As she did this, it became easier to focus on her client rather than on her worries about being fired. As she learned to steady herself, and practice being receptive to whatever arose in her awareness, she began to talk less and listen more. Things began to shift. Clients appreciated her ability to listen to them and began to request her. As her confidence in her skills increased she settled into her job. Her boss, realizing that Amy was a hardworking and loyal employee, began to relax as well.

In their research on depression, Williams et al. (2007) have explored how what is happening in our minds affects our bodies, often without our conscious awareness: "When a negative thought or image arises in the mind, there will be a sense of contraction, tightening or bracing in the body somewhere" (p. 25). If we interrupt this unconscious habitual response, we may be able to stop a downward spiral, as Amy learned to do.

The following practice builds on the foundation of concentration. It moves beyond attention to sensations to include awareness of the mind's response to sensations, and thereby offers another transition from concentration practice to open monitoring. Before teaching this to patients, it is best if they first have some ability to anchor in sounds, touch points, or breathing.

AWARENESS OF SENSATION

- Start by sitting comfortably. Spend a few moments tuning into sounds. No need to chase them, just allow them to come and go. If it is comfortable, bring your attention to the breath. Notice where you feel it most strongly (nostrils, chest, belly) and if you like, silently note "rising, falling" or "in, out" as the breath enters and leaves the body.

- Keep your attention on either sounds or the breath until a physical sensation is strong enough to distract you. Notice what it is that takes you away and make a mental note of it. Don't worry about using the precise word. Pressure, throbbing, burning, itching, stabbing—whatever it is, pleasant or unpleasant, allow it to arise and pass away.

- Notice your reaction to the sensation. Do you want to hold on to it, push it away, or ignore it?

- Bring kind and careful attention to all sensations. If you experience pain, see if you can open to it. We often think of pain as solid and unremitting, but with careful attention we notice that pain arises and then subsides. A stab, then a respite. Pressure, burning, then rest.

- Notice what happens when you observe any discomfort. Can you notice different strands or threads of sensation?

- See what your mind might be adding to any pain or emotional discomfort. Do you cringe in fear? Are you fighting it? Blaming or berating yourself for having it? Worrying that it will get worse or never stop?

- After a while, return to the breath or sounds. Remind yourself that there's no need to dwell on the discomfort. See if you can find a balance between exploring other sensations and returning to your anchor.

- Remember that both pain and pleasure are impermanent. Let them come and go, without grasping, avoiding, or trying to fix them. End your meditation by anchoring your attention in sounds, the touch points, or the breath. Try to remain mindful during your next activity.

CLINICAL ILLUSTRATION: SHIFTING THE RELATIONSHIP WITH PAIN

Monique entered treatment overwhelmed with the chronic pain of fibromyalgia. She had been suffering for years and had grown increasingly frustrated and angry when doctors told her it was "all in her head." She became more isolated, stopped working, and spent most of her time sleeping or watching TV. "I'm not a nut case, really, I'm not," she insisted. After a careful evaluation, the therapist suggested mindfulness practice. Monique was dismissive. "I really don't see how gazing at my navel is going to make any difference," she challenged. "This is ridiculous. You can't help me. You're just like the other quacks. I'm not going to waste my time."

Monique's therapist took a few deep breaths and noticed her own anger emerging as she considered how to respond. She thought of a story in which a man reaches out to pat a dog and the dog responds by biting his hand. It turns out that the dog's foot, which was covered by leaves, is caught in a trap. Realizing that Monique was caught in pain helped her therapist not take the attack personally and respond in kind by angrily escorting her out the door. "Research actually shows that meditation can help a lot with chronic pain problems. When we are more focused in the present and don't anticipate or tense up against pain, the experience of pain is diminished. Meditation also helps us not get caught up in our negative thoughts about the pain" (see Siegel, 2013). Monique rolled her eyes. "OK, I'll try it. I guess I have nothing to lose, but I don't see how it's going to help," she sighed. In spite of her initial hostility, Monique resonated with the practice of breathing and liked the challenge of counting her breaths. With daily practice of 15 minutes a day for several weeks, she noticed a difference and began to feel less overwhelmed by the pain. In the beginning, Monique thought of her pain as constant and unrelenting. In session, guided by her therapist, she began to explore one ache at a time. "My knees hurt, my feet hurt, my back hurts," she reported, "everything hurts all the time." "Can you locate any places where you don't feel discomfort?" her therapist asked. "My ears, my pinky finger," Monique responded. "Good," the therapist replied, "notice where there is pain, as well as where you might find ease."

As she learned to become aware of her bodily sensations, Monique was surprised to find that her daily aches, chills, and pain actually came in waves. When she was young, she had been an avid surfer and skier. While Monique originally felt that her body had betrayed her, she eventually realized that she could draw upon her earlier athletic skills as she experimented with riding the waves of discomfort.

As she practiced, Monique became aware of subtle sensations and was able to identify what made them worse. One morning she had a pain in her foot. Within a nanosecond, she found herself wondering if she would be able to walk that day. She then worried that she had broken a bone. Suddenly, she was envisioning surgery and wondering how she would get around on crutches and who would take her to the hospital. She laughed at how quickly she had gone into catastrophic thinking, aware of the distress her mind had added to the problem.

Monique's insight was informed by the Buddhist parable of the two arrows, which her therapist had shared with her. This well-known teaching story explains the difference between those who are trained in mindfulness and those who are not. When the latter feel a painful sensation, they not only experience the initial physical pain but also the mental suffering that soon follows. So it is like being struck by two arrows instead of just one. Monique joked that she had added the third, fourth, and fifth arrows. "I never saw this before. I just thought I was preparing myself for the worst, that it was actually helpful to think this way."

Noticing that the pain wasn't constant and that there were moments of respite motivated her. Monique began venturing out of her apartment and, on the suggestion of a friend, enrolled in a tai chi class. While she continued to experience pain, she also learned to navigate through it. She no longer felt like it was running her life. Monique became a fan of Mark Twain's famous line: "I am a very old man and have suffered a great many misfortunes, most of which never happened."

MINDFULNESS OF EMOTIONS

Becoming aware of emotions in the body is a practical way to locate and feel them, and like sensations, allow them to come and go. As we move into what can be more challenging terrain for patients, the body provides a place to ground and anchor difficult feelings so they can be worked with effectively, rather than become overwhelming. This practice can help establish greater balance and perspective during the storms of life.

AWARENESS OF EMOTIONS IN THE BODY

- Start by sitting comfortably, eyes either closed or half open. Spend a few minutes listening to the sounds around you, noticing the touch points, or the rise and fall of the breath. Let yourself feel the comfort of your anchor.
- If you like, try a body sweep. Notice places of tension, discomfort, or holding.
- See if you can identify the "emotional weather" in your internal landscape. Are there feelings of anger . . . sadness . . . anxiety . . . fear?
- Return to your anchor. See which emotional "winds" carry you away. Make whatever carries you away the object of your attention.
- See if you can locate where the emotion resides in your body. Tune in—is there pressure in your chest? Clenching of the jaw? Tightness in the shoulders? Do you feel a pit in your stomach? Is your pulse racing? Does your head ache? Are your eyes heavy? Bring careful attention and kind curiosity to what you are feeling and noticing.
- Be with the emotion in a gentle way. Notice if you start to

criticize or berate yourself. Notice if you start to disconnect. What takes you away?

- Once you've noticed where the emotion resides in your body, check the rest of your body to see what is happening. Does your chest collapse in response to fear in your stomach?

- Try bringing the warmth of your hand to the place where the emotion is most intense. Invite this place to soften and relax. Try breathing into this discomfort. Sometimes just becoming aware of the emotion in a friendly and curious way can help. Don't struggle or resist. Just notice it and allow it to be.

- If you start to feel overwhelmed, lost, or distracted, simply return to the breath, sounds, or touch points. Notice any judgments the mind adds on, letting them come and go.

- When you are ready, take a breath, wiggle your fingers and toes, stretch, and open your eyes if they have been closed. Try to remain mindful during your next activity.

CLINICAL ILLUSTRATION: NOTHING BUT HEARTACHE

Emily, a graduate student in her 20s, was having a difficult time. Her boyfriend of many years had just broken up with her and she was heartbroken. Some days she stayed in bed without showering or eating. She felt that she couldn't live without him and at times wanted to die. For the first time in her life she couldn't sleep and had no appetite. She couldn't concentrate on her school work, spent hours each day in tears, and worried that she was going crazy. "I don't think this pain will ever end. I'm afraid that I'll need to be institutionalized."

Emily had a beginning meditation practice and wanted to see if more mindfulness practice could help. When she tuned into her body, it seemed that her pain occupied every inch of her being. As she stayed with it, she experienced most of her emotion in her stomach. It felt like all the wind had been knocked out of her. She put a hand on her stomach, feeling comforted by the soothing touch and warmth. She found that breathing into the sharp pain helped soften it, giving her some space—like a brief break in a storm, as she put it. She became curious and wanted to explore this more. Her therapist taught her a variation on *Awareness of Emotions in the Body* used by Tara Brach (2013) in which she was invited to find her undefended 2-year-old belly. This brought her back to the time when her family was still intact and her father still lived at home. This was when, as she put it, "My world was still steady."

She had seen her mother collapse and be hospitalized for severe depression after being deserted by Emily's father. She did not want to become a "mess" like her mother. "I'm in school so I can have a better life; I'm not going to blow this," she said. This determination helped her practice meditation through tears and sleepless nights. She felt that it provided some scaffolding so she could "get a grip" and begin to climb out of her despair.

Over weeks and months of practice and therapy, there were more breaks in the storm clouds. Emily began to realize that her heartache was not permanent, that like all things, it would pass. "I really thought that my life was over once James left. And then I realized that I still had a life without him. I'm lonely a lot. I hate weekends. I miss sex and being held. But, I found a resilience that I never knew I had, one that I'd never seen in my family, where it was one disaster after another." No one was going to take this away from her. As Emily stabilized and was able to sleep, eat, and return to school, she began to explore her feelings around her father's leaving and see the ways this early and profound loss was being reenacted.

The Power of Labeling

Labeling is a well-researched meditation practice. Creswell, Way, Eisenberger, and Lieberman (2007) found that in the process of labeling our experience, we deactivate the amygdala (the brain's alarm center) and access the medial prefrontal cortex, thus moving out of a state of reactivity into a place where we can reestablish balance and find perspective. Meditation teacher Joseph Goldstein (1993) clarifies the method in a way that can be very helpful to patients. He writes: "Labeling, like putting a frame around a picture, helps you recognize the object more clearly and gives greater focus and precision to your observation" (p. 35). The clinical implications are enormous. This practice can be used for many disorders and is suitable for a wide array of patients who are struggling with disturbing feelings.

LABELING EMOTIONS

- Start by sitting comfortably, eyes either closed or partially open. Take a few deep breaths, or if you prefer, bring your attention to the sounds around you.

- Spend a few moments connecting with your anchor. When you are taken away by an emotion, note what the emotion is. With an attitude of warmth and acceptance, label the emotion. For example, note, "worry, worry, worry." Don't obsess about getting the label exactly right. It doesn't need to be precise to be effective.

- See where you find this emotion in your body. Allow yourself to simply be with it.

- Notice the attitude you bring to this practice. Are you yelling at yourself when you notice "anger, anger, anger"? Are you telling yourself that you're a bad person for having this emotion? See if you can label with kindness, warmth, and acceptance.

- If the emotion becomes too intense and you start to get overwhelmed or lost in it, simply return to your anchor.

- There is no need to hold on to or analyze the emotion. Let it rise and fall away. No need to go into the history or story behind the emotion either. Label it and let it go.

- Label the emotions with as much warmth and kindness as possible. If you feel that negative emotions don't deserve kindness, label this as well. Be open to pleasant emotions and label them too.

- Continue to alternate between labeling the emotions and grounding with your anchor. When you're ready, take a few deep breaths, wiggle your fingers and toes, stretch, and open your eyes if they have been closed. Try to continue to be aware of your emotional reactions as you move into your next activity.

Available in audio at *www.sittingtogether.com*.

CLINICAL ILLUSTRATION: WHAT LIES BENEATH

Fernando was a single man in his 40s. He had never married because he had not found the "perfect woman." He had a meditation practice that was an important part of his life, but he entered treatment because he was concerned about the time he spent on Internet pornography and the money he spent on prostitutes. On the surface he was a respectable professional and he felt ashamed and sullied by his secret life. The problem, as he saw it, was learning to control his "excessive sexuality."

Fernando's therapist suggested that labeling emotions might help him to gain perspective on his sexual feelings and behavior. As he began to practice labeling he was very aware of lust. He practiced noting "lust, lust, lust" with a tone of kindness rather than disgust. This was a challenge because it took him back to childhood, where his religious family condemned his masturbation, calling it repulsive. As he began to bring interest rather than judgment to his sexuality, he was surprised to find layers of unexplored feelings. First he encountered sadness, which he labeled and allowed himself to feel. Underneath this feeling he encountered intense rage, accompanied by images of physically attacking and punishing his family. It was hard to experience this and he labeled it "rage, rage, rage" as kindly as he could. When this emotion had passed, he became aware of a profound loneliness that dated back as far as he could remember. "No one in my family ever showed warmth or affection," he recalled, "and there was very little physical contact." Fernando realized that underneath what he thought was excessive sexual desire was in fact a deep loneliness that he had never acknowledged. He also saw that part of the allure of prostitutes was being with someone who would simply hold and comfort him. He and his therapist went on to explore how this longing had shaped so many of his life choices.

While Fernando was disheartened to realize that his obsession had such deep roots, he also realized that it was never too late to "turn on the light." This is true for all our patients. As Sharon Salzberg (2011) writes, "When you flip the switch in that attic, it doesn't matter whether it's been dark for ten minutes, ten years, or ten decades" (p. 129).

This practice can be deepened by not only labeling emotions ("lonely, lonely, lonely"), but thoughts as well. Fernando practiced labeling this way: "A thought that no one wants to be with me." "A thought that I am disgusting." "A thought that I am unlovable." While it may be challenging, it is important to use kindness when noticing the judging mind. Fernando practiced letting his thoughts come and go, like clouds moving across the sky. It was also helpful that his therapist pointed out that the feeling of the moment wouldn't last forever and wasn't the totality of who he is. As the poet Rilke (1905/2005) phrased it, "no feeling is final" (p. 171).

A useful variation of labeling involves taking the self out of the equation when identifying thoughts and emotions. As discussed in Chapters 1 and 3, when we observe thoughts and feelings as impersonal events, they become less overwhelming. Saying, "I am angry" can easily give rise to, "and I've always been angry, and I always will be and this will never change and it all goes back to when my angry father was abusive toward me." Instead, we can try saying, "Anger is arising." With this impersonal framing of the emotion, it is easier to let it pass rather than holding on to it or owning it as a defining quality that will always be true. Joseph Goldstein (1993) has his students add the neutral thought, "And the sky is blue." He writes, "By adding it to the end of every judgment, I got a sense of what it would be like to let the judgment go through my mind in just the same way 'the sky is blue' goes through" (p. 65). Many patients like this technique, as it takes the charge out of the feeling, making it easier to let it pass and seeing it as part of the nature of things, part of the vastness of human experience.

PUTTING IT ALL TOGETHER

The following exercise combines the earlier open monitoring meditations to shed light on sensations, thoughts, feelings, and behavior, revealing how they interact and inform one another. It is inspired by the teaching of Michael Grady at Cambridge Insight Meditation Center.

FINDING THE PATTERN

- Start by sitting comfortably, eyes either open or closed. Find your posture of dignity. Spend a few moments establishing concentration, either with sounds, the touch points, or the breath.
- Bring your attention to the sensations in your body. Do a quick body sweep to become aware of places of tension, tightness, or discomfort.
- Stay with one sensation until you get pulled away by a thought or emotion. Let this mental content become the object of your meditation. Bring your full awareness to it. Be curious.
- Bring kind and gentle attention to the thought or emotion. If judgment and criticism arise, note this, and if you like, gently label it. Keep watching the thoughts and feelings. If you get overwhelmed, return to your anchor.
- See if you can discern sequences. For example, is a sensation

of tightness in the chest followed by a feeling of panic? Does the panic then trigger a thought, such as "I have to get out of here"? Stay with your experience, be gentle, and take your time. Bring your attention, curiosity, and intelligence to the process.

• See if you can note if behavior is part of the sequence and tied to thoughts or feelings. Explore how this comes together for you.

• Try to continue to be aware of the sequences of sensations, emotions, thoughts, and behavior as you move into your next activity.

CLINICAL ILLUSTRATION: A NEW PAIR OF GLASSES

Tamara was a woman in her late 30s who had left a secure job to become a yoga teacher. Her husband was a graphic designer who had recently lost his job and was unable to find a new position. They had a young child in elementary school.

Tamara entered therapy to deal with her increasing panic. It was hard to make ends meet and the bills were piling up. She was also feeling like a fraud. She had to play the role of a smiling, mellow, calm, yoga teacher when in fact she was having panic attacks and drinking Scotch and wine every night to fall asleep. She was berating herself for giving up her stable job, calling herself a hypocrite. When she tried to meditate she found that she was yelling at herself, "You stupid, impractical idiot," in a voice that mimicked her father's. She also noticed that she was getting increasingly angry with her husband for his passivity.

Tamara's therapist suggested that she try to notice the sequence of her sensations, thoughts, emotions, and behaviors during her meditation. As she took up this practice, she began to notice the sequence of these events in her life more broadly. In therapy she became aware of a tightness and clenching in her chest, a sensation she often experienced in the middle of the night. This sensation was followed by the recurrent thought, "We can't make it. If Joe doesn't get a job we'll have to move in with my parents. I'd rather die." This thought was often accompanied by a feeling of dizziness and a racing pulse. At this point in the sequence, Tamara realized that she would reach for the Scotch and then eat ice cream and chocolate cookies. After indulging, she would criticize her husband for watching TV or checking Facebook rather than finding work.

When Tamara noticed this pattern, she said that she felt like she had been given a new pair of glasses. She recalled a time in grade school when a teacher noticed that she couldn't read the board. When she got corrective lenses, she was stunned by how different the world looked. She had assumed that trees, buildings, signs, and people were supposed to be blurry. She hadn't realized that objects had distinct forms and shapes, sharp edges, and vibrant colors. "Everything had been in soft focus and it all merged together. Clarity was a new experience. My perception of the world totally changed."

As Tamara became aware of her mind's sequences she found ways to interrupt the downward spirals. She practiced working with her anchor as soon as she felt the tightness in her chest. She tried feeling the soles of her feet and doing some yoga instead of reaching for the Scotch. As she was able to acknowledge what was happening, she realized that she was angry. This broke through her denial and she began to talk to her husband rather than yell at him. They entered couple therapy to renegotiate their marriage and find a less stressful way to live.

Tamara learned that she could create some space between her emotions and her habitual responses. Difficult feelings and negative thoughts are part of everyone's experience. Without awareness, they can hijack our behavior. If we notice these patterns on the meditation cushion, however, we are more likely to notice and interrupt them in the rest of our lives.

The benefits of mindfulness practice appear to be dose related, so it helps to make an effort to do informal mindfulness practices through-out the day—being aware of our body when we walk to the bus or car, noticing sensations in the body when we cook dinner, bringing attention to emotions and the underlying patterns as the day unfolds. We can label thoughts and emotions and bring awareness to sequences during these activities much as during formal practice.

IT'S OK TO LOSE IT

Don't worry if you or your patients get reactive and unmindful. As Christina Feldman (2001) writes: "Mindfulness is neither difficult nor complex; *remembering* to be mindful is the great challenge." (p. 167) The aim of mindfulness practice is to train our attention so we become more aware of our inner and outer landscape, and forgetting is part of the process. "The moment we recognize that we've lost mindfulness, we have already regained it; that recognition is its essence. We can begin again" (Salzberg, 2011, p. 105).

CHAPTER SIX

Loving-Kindness and Compassion Practice

Engaging the Heart

> Compassion is not a luxury. It is a necessity for human beings to survive.
> —The Dalai Lama (in Halifax, 2012)

Loving-kindness and compassion can grow and flourish in the fertile ground that has been prepared by concentration and open monitoring or mindfulness. When we practice gathering our attention and returning again and again, without judgment or criticism, our mind gradually becomes more accepting and less reactive. As Joseph Goldstein (1993) puts it, with time [our] "meditation develops a tremendous tenderness of heart . . . that transforms the way we relate to ourselves and others. We begin to feel more deeply, and the depth of feeling becomes the wellspring of compassion" (p. 147).

Loving-kindness and compassion open the heart in slightly different ways. While loving-kindness involves wishing others well, compassion involves, in the words of psychologist Paul Gilbert (2009c), who developed compassion-focused therapy, the "suffering of oneself and of other living beings, coupled with the wish and effort to relieve it" (p. xiii). Compassion is therefore action oriented. As Thich Nhat Hanh teaches, it is something we do, not just an idea or a feeling. Compassion literally means to "suffer with" (Siegel & Germer, 2012, p. 12) and is therefore by its nature relational. It connects us with others and challenges our assumptions of separation and aloneness. Compassion is a fundamental human capacity described by religious traditions throughout the ages (Armstrong, 2010) that helps us become aware of our common humanity, the understanding that we all are vulnerable to heartbreak, loss, illness, and death.

For therapists, compassion is a lifeline that helps us remain resilient in the face of suffering. As Sharon Salzberg (1997) writes: "The state of compassion is whole and sustaining; the compassionate mind is not broken or shattered by facing states of suffering. It is spacious and resilient" (p. 133). Compassion is therefore an essential component of psychotherapy for ourselves and our patients (Germer & Siegel, 2012).

Like concentration and mindfulness, loving-kindness and compassion are also skills that can be learned and cultivated. Through neurobiological research and the work of scholars and clinicians, we are beginning to understand the dramatic benefits of training in these abilities (Davidson, 2012; Fredrickson, 2012; Germer, 2009; Gilbert, 2009a; Germer & Siegel, 2012; Neff, 2011; Neff & Germer, 2013). And we are discovering that compassion in particular is probably a curative factor in most forms of psychotherapy (Shapiro & Carlson, 2009; Hölzel et al., 2011).

Loving-kindness and compassion practices help us transform the way we treat ourselves and others. By paying attention to our thoughts, feelings, and actions we open our hearts to loving ourselves for who we are, with all our imperfections. And as we learn to care for ourselves, we are better able to see people in all their complexity. With training we might be "inclined to wish them well instead of becoming irritated, to let go of past hurts . . . to offer a friendly gesture to someone we might previously have ignored, or find a better way to deal with a difficult person" (Salzberg, 2011, p. 16). While concentration and open monitoring enable us to see the distinction between our experience and the story we're creating about it, loving-kindness and compassion have "the power to change our story" (p. 167).

While enormously beneficial, cultivating compassion in particular can be challenging. It is difficult for most of us to open fully to suffering, no less to our wishes to alleviate it. Buddhist meditation traditions have evolved a stepwise approach to this challenge. Once a certain degree of concentration has been developed, practitioners work to cultivate loving-kindness (*metta* in Pali) before focusing on compassion per se. Since loving-kindness involves wishing ourselves and others well, but does not necessarily include attention to suffering (Siegel & Germer, 2012), it can serve as a good foundation for compassion practice.

Loving-kindness is traditionally cultivated by using a series of phrases that express kind wishes for ourselves and others. These phrases include variations on the following:

> *May I be safe.*
> *May I be happy.*
> *May I be healthy.*
> *May I be peaceful.*
> *May I be free from suffering.*
> *May I live with ease.*

The "may I" is not said in a spirit of begging or asking permission, but expresses a wish or intention for ourselves and others. These phrases can also be simplified by just silently repeating some of the key words, such as *"safe . . . healthy . . . ease"* or *"happy . . . peaceful . . . free from suffering."* In loving-kindness practice, we try to bring our full attention, energy, and intelligence to each phrase. These phrases can bring needed nutrients to the dry, exhausted, or frozen places within.

Depending on a person's religious and cultural background, these practices can feel a lot like prayer. Sometimes secular individuals will therefore feel uncomfortable trying them, finding them to be "preachy" or "too formulaic." If that's the case, emphasizing that we're working to connect to and strengthen a feeling—not asking an external entity for assistance—can be helpful. For those who don't like using phrases, we have found that using a visual image of safety, health, peace, and ease can work just as well. People with a more theistic background will often find themselves asking God to bring well-being to themselves or others, as in supplicant prayer. For them, a more religious framework can be effective for cultivating loving-kindness. Here is a beginning loving-kindness exercise suitable for most patients.

OFFERING LOVING-KINDNESS TO ONESELF

- Start by sitting comfortably with eyes either open or closed. Spend a few minutes with your anchor—either sounds, touch points, or the breath.
- Let yourself settle, noting any tension or discomfort in the body. Invite it to soften.
- Begin by directing kindness toward yourself with some of the traditional phrases: *May I be safe. May I be healthy. May I live with ease.* Or perhaps, *May I be happy. May I be peaceful. May I be free from suffering.* Choose whichever of these phrases, or others of your own, that evoke a feeling of soothing loving-kindness.
- Say the phrases silently to yourself, finding a rhythm that feels comfortable. See if you can open to each phrase. If one phrase speaks to you, it is fine to stay with that for a while.
- Feel that each phrase contains an essential vitamin that you need or imagine them as a gentle, irrigating rain falling on parched soil.
- Try the experiment of conjuring an image that evokes safety, health, peace, and ease. If it seems to enrich your sense of loving-kindness, continue visualizing the image.
- If the mind wanders, no problem. Return to the phrases or image, letting them become your anchor.
- When you are ready, take a deep breath, stretch, and open your eyes if they have been closed. See if you can carry an attitude of loving-kindness into your next activity.

Available in audio at *www.sittingtogether.com*.

CLINICAL ILLUSTRATION: "GOOD MORNING, HEARTACHE"

Dylan was a musician in his late 30s. The last few years had been particularly difficult. The band he created and that had formed his identity for over a decade had fallen apart and it was increasingly hard to find work on his own. His wife, tired of his late nights and his use of recreational drugs, had left. Dylan found himself at loose ends, waking up anxious, heartbroken, and bereft. The Billie Holiday standard "Good Morning Heartache" spoke to him, expressing his feelings of a ruined life and dashed hopes.

Longing for some kindness and wanting something beyond

medication to help him with his despair, Dylan attended a workshop on compassion at his local meditation center. Like many people, initially he found it difficult to send loving-kindness to himself because he felt undeserving. So his therapist suggested that he experiment with first sending kindness and care to a "benefactor," a traditional form of practice (see the *Compassionate Being* exercise, page 112). Dylan chose his grandmother, as she had been a supportive and comforting figure, especially when his mother had been hospitalized for a psychotic break.

For the first few weeks nothing useful seemed to be happening. In fact, Dylan got angry with himself because he kept falling asleep (this often happens in the early stages of practice as we slow down and notice our exhaustion and sleep deprivation). His therapist empathically noted that the end of a marriage and the demise of a career are major losses to process, and fatigue is natural when things fall apart. She suggested that he continue with the meditation, but try standing if he noticed he was getting sleepy. Dylan liked this variation and persisted with the practice.

Slowly, he felt the practice began to make a "dent" in his morning heartache. As he worked with the phrases, they become comforting and stabilizing. He called them his reminder of the "possibility of sanity." They were useful in rush hour traffic, helping him calm his road rage. Sometimes he just stayed with one phrase when he felt especially anxious or agitated. He felt that *May I be safe* helped him get a little "traction" and perspective. The phrases also became a tool to help him manage his volatile emotions in more intimate interactions. After one particularly contentious fight with his wife over dividing possessions, he was able to soothe himself and prevent a binge by adapting a sequence of phrases from meditation teacher and psychologist Sylvia Boorstein (2007): *Dude, this is a moment of pain. Everyone has suffering. Relax, take a deep breath. We will figure this out.* As Dylan began to pick up the pieces of his life, loving-kindness practice helped him find stable ground.

As Jack Kornfield (1993) points out, we cannot avoid difficulties or mistakes, but we can learn "the art of making mistakes wakefully, bringing to them the transformative power of our heart" (p. 72). It is inevitable that we will confront our own limitations. One Zen master described life as "one mistake after another"—and it is from these mistakes that we learn and grow. Along similar lines Kornfield notes that to "live life is to make a succession of errors. Understanding this can bring us great ease and forgiveness for ourselves and others" (p. 72).

BRINGING COMPASSION TO THE BODY

Body Scan is an essential component of MBSR (Kabat-Zinn, 1990), the secular, systematic program widely used to introduce mindfulness into health care practice. Neff and Germer (2013) have converted this practice into a compassion-building exercise in their 8-week course on mindful self-compassion (MSC). The following is a further adaptation geared toward individual therapy. While in MBSR it is taught starting with the feet and moving up through the body, in individual therapy some patients find it more effective to start with the head and move down. Meditation teachers suggest that starting with the feet can help with grounding, whereas starting with the head and eyes can help soften tension. Both are effective: Feel free to experiment with what works for the patients in your practice. While this practice is traditionally taught lying down, it can also be done sitting upright or standing.

COMPASSIONATE BODY SCAN

- Find a comfortable position either sitting or lying down.
- Take a few moments to settle and center yourself, using the practice of sounds, touch points, or the breath. Come into the present moment. Let go of regrets about the past or worries about the future.
- Bring attention to the head, eyes, and jaw, allowing any tension to soften. Rest here for a few moments, taking it all in. If you notice pain or emotional discomfort, bring kind and loving attention to that part of your body.
- Move into the neck and throat, allowing them to soften, bringing soothing attention to any tightness or discomfort.
- Continue down into the shoulders and chest, filling your body with kindness. Notice any discomfort and invite it to soften. Bring a gentle and kind attention to any pain or emotion. Don't fight or resist, let it be as it is. Bring attention to both of your arms simultaneously, from the upper arms down to the fingertips. If this is a difficult time for you, let your hand rest on your heart, feeling this soothing and comforting touch.
- Continue with the belly, back, and pelvis, bringing kind, compassionate attention to every part of your body. If difficult feelings arise, either return to your breath or try

repeating some of the loving-kindness phrases: *May I be safe. May I be healthy. May I be peaceful. May I live with ease.* Or try your own variations, such as *May I be free from inner and outer harm* or *May I love myself completely, just as I am.* If you like, you can simplify the sequence to just the key words: *safe . . . healthy . . . peaceful . . . ease.* Let these words land, receive them. Let them nourish you.

- If you come up against a strong dislike of any part of the body, try saying in the kindest tone you can: *May I love and accept my body just as it is. May I bring kindness and compassion to this body.*

- Bring kind attention to the thighs, knees, ankles, and feet, appreciating all that your body does and how hard it works for you. If you get distracted, return to the phrases or the breath. If you feel overwhelmed by a feeling associated with a particular area, you can bypass this part of your body and return to it when you are ready.

- End with compassion for your entire body, with all its scars, imperfections, discomforts, or illnesses. See if you can appreciate this body, loving it as it is right now.

- When you are ready, especially if you are lying down, stretch, wiggle fingers and toes, rotate wrists and ankles, turn to one side, and slowly get up. See if you can carry an attitude of self-compassion into your next activity.

CLINICAL ILLUSTRATION: BRINGING KINDNESS TO THE BODY

Jessica was a high school student stressed out by the pressure of SATs and caught between her parents who were going through a bitter divorce. Her boyfriend had been a source of support, but when he started dating someone else it was more than she could take. She began cutting herself, first discreetly but then more dramatically. Her parents, preoccupied with their own drama, didn't notice, but an attentive coach did and helped Jessica find help.

In her first few therapy sessions, Jessica mostly just wept. As she began to feel more comfortable, she talked about how hard things were at home and how stressful things were at school. She was taking yoga in gym class and really liked the meditation and relaxation at the end. To incorporate this into therapy, her therapist started with the practice of *Touch Points* (see Chapter 4, page 70). She utilized this technique during exams and stressful moments, finding it especially useful when she ran into her ex-boyfriend with his new girlfriend. After these encounters, however, she would still go home and cut herself in the privacy of her bathroom. She described it as a "release"—a way to discharge the pain and stress of her life.

While Jessica found the *Touch Points* practice relaxing and enjoyed it in therapy, she was unable to practice on her own, often "forgetting" to do it. When she and her therapist looked at this in treatment, Jessica complained that the practice took too much of her time. Her therapist shared an insight that had helped when she struggled with the same issue: "One of my teachers once told me that we didn't start from scratch each time we practiced; we could pick up where we left off." Jessica smiled. "I like that. It makes it less difficult, like it isn't so much work." Later, when she started wearing summer clothes and the scars from months of cutting became more visible, she was finally ready to address her secret. She began to practice compassionate body scan in treatment, bringing kind attention to every part of her body. After weeks of working to appreciate and be kind to her body, she was less inclined to bring a knife or razor blade to her skin. Of course, there were still bad days when she cut. At these times, instead of becoming mired in feelings of shame and guilt, she and her therapist worked on maintaining loving-kindness and compassion, adding the phrases: *May I be kind to myself. May I not cause physical harm. May I be safe and protected. May I love myself just as I am.* She found that she didn't need to dwell on her destructive acts and could start again.

Gradually her life began to stabilize. The divorce was settled and issues around custody were resolved. Jessica was accepted by a college that she wanted to attend. While the urge to cut didn't disappear entirely, she felt that she had more options and resources. Although she hadn't been able to establish a daily practice, she reported that she was able to use the meditations when she needed them. By practicing the body scan and using loving-kindness and compassion phrases, she found that she could interrupt the desire to cut and instead call a friend, listen to music, go for a run, practice yoga, or write about her feelings in a journal. In difficult moments, she used what Germer and Neff call a "self-compassion break" (Germer, 2009; Neff, 2011; Neff & Germer, 2013): She would stop, put a hand on her heart and say, *Jessica, this is a moment of suffering. All people suffer. Life is hard sometimes. Just let me feel this. Let me be kind to myself. Let me care for my body.*

BRINGING COMPASSION TO EATING

Many patients have difficulty controlling their eating and suffer from self-critical judgments about their food intake. Mindful eating is a core

practice in MBSR that we have adapted to include eating with compassion (see Fain, 2011). This can be useful for a range of eating disorders,
including anorexia, bulimia, and overeating. For this exercise, you can
use raisins, dried cherries or cranberries, or fresh fruit—whatever is
most comfortable and convenient. Pick three fruits of the same variety
for this exercise.

COMPASSIONATE EATING

- Start by sitting comfortably, eyes either open or closed,
  feeling the support of the chair.

- Give yourself a few minutes to settle and come into the body.
  Use the practice of sounds, touch points, or your breath to
  come into the present moment.

- Open your eyes if they were closed. Put the three fruits in
  front of you on a napkin or plate. Just notice the fruit, taking
  in color, shape, shadow, and the play of light.

- Pick up one piece of fruit. Gently hold it between your
  fingers. Be aware of what it feels like. Notice its texture.
  Turn it over in your hand. Look at it as if you had never seen
  it before, bringing to your seeing the quality of "beginner's
  mind."

- Bring it to your nose. Notice its smell. Bring it to your lips.
  What does it feel like? Be aware of the temperature and other
  qualities.

- Place the fruit in your mouth, letting it rest on your tongue.
  Wait a moment before starting to chew. Allow your mouth
  to respond. Be aware of all the sensations.

- As you begin to chew, notice what happens. Do this slowly
  and mindfully. Be aware of the taste and the sensations of
  chewing. Allow yourself to enjoy this simple act of eating,
  chewing, and swallowing.

- Pause for a moment, and begin sending loving-kindness
  or compassion toward yourself. You might silently repeat
  phrases such as *May I love and care for my body, May I feed
  myself, May I nourish myself.* Choose whatever phrases you find
  comforting and nurturing.

- Repeat this process with the second and then third piece of fruit. See what you notice each time. Allow yourself to savor the food and to nourish yourself.

- When you are ready, take a few deep breaths, wiggle fingers and toes, and stretch. See if you can carry an attitude of mindful nurturing into your next activity.

CLINICAL ILLUSTRATION: "MAY I LEARN TO CARE FOR MY BODY"

Nancy had struggled with overeating her entire life. In her 50 years, she had tried almost every well-known diet—Atkins, South Beach, Weight Watchers—plus more fad diets than she cared to discuss. In fact, she claimed that she had been on a perpetual diet since age 13 when her brother had called her "fat." She had tried hypnosis to curb her cravings for donuts and ice cream, but nothing worked for long. She read about a book on mindfulness and weight loss in her favorite women's magazine and signed up for a course in meditation. Her teacher suggested individual therapy as well.

She began working with a therapist. As they practiced compassionate eating together, Nancy realized that she had never really tasted a blueberry before. She was eating, as she put it, "on auto pilot," stuffing herself without awareness that she was even eating. She joked that sometimes she didn't even come up for air.

As she slowed down and began to really taste her food, she realized that by the third spoonful of cookie dough ice cream she had stopped tasting it. Once she saw this, she experimented with stopping after three spoonfuls rather than finishing the entire pint. She started slowly, making small changes in her eating habits. Five cups of coffee with cream and three sugars were whittled down to one; three glasses of supersized soda gave way to water; take-out fried chicken, pizza, and burgers with large fries evolved into healthier options.

As Nancy used compassionate eating as a daily meditation, she repeated the phrases: *May I love and care for my body. May I feed myself. May I nourish myself.* She realized that much of her overeating was a way to stuff her emotions and self-soothe. She began to talk about childhood sexual abuse and the ways she used her weight to become less attractive to her abuser: "I got so fat that no one would ever want me." She had felt soiled and degraded most of her life. She experienced her body as disgusting, repulsive—she was so dissociated from it that it didn't feel like her body. As she and her therapist explored the memories of abuse, Nancy added the phrases: *May I be free of hatred, disgust, and regret. May I be free of the wounds of my childhood.*

Bringing compassion to eating helped Nancy begin to reclaim her body and start to heal from her trauma. In addition to her individual therapy, she joined a group of abuse survivors. "I'll never be skinny," she noted, "but I refuse to perpetuate the abuse by eating until I make myself sick."

TAKING COMPASSION FROM THE
MEDITATION CUSHION INTO THE WORLD

The next practice is a variation on walking meditation taught by Sharon Salzberg (2011). It can be practiced any time we're out in the world, supplementing formal loving-kindness practices, or when more formal meditation practices might be overwhelming.

BRINGING COMPASSION INTO DAILY LIFE

- Start by standing comfortably, finding your balance and taking a few breaths to center and ground.
- Next silently repeat these or other loving-kindness phrases: *May I be safe. May I be healthy. May I be peaceful. May I live with ease.*
- Begin to walk at a comfortable pace, saying these phrases as you move. If you like, coordinate them with either your breath or your footsteps. As you walk by people or animals, wish them well, silently saying, *May you be safe. May you be healthy. May you be peaceful. May you live with ease.*
- There is no need to tell others what you are doing; just silently offer them kindness as you pass by. Don't feel the need to send loving-kindness and compassion to everyone you pass. It's fine to choose just a few.
- If this feels uncomfortable, or if you are going through a difficult time, return to sending loving-kindness to just yourself for a while. Then, once you feel ready, experiment again with sending loving-kindness and compassion to all living beings that pass by—dogs, cats, birds. You can even include trees and flowers.
- You can take this practice into places that scare you— highways, doctors' offices, airplanes, elevators, crowded spaces. If you get overwhelmed, return to your breath and send loving-kindness and compassion to yourself.

CLINICAL ILLUSTRATION: A FEAR WORSE THAN DEATH

A young teacher named Carmen entered therapy to work with her severe fear of public speaking. She would become physically ill, shaking and vomiting before teaching a class. To her, public speaking was worse than death. This fear had plagued her since childhood, when she froze at a school play and ran offstage in tears. Her internist had prescribed beta blockers, which helped, but she wanted to find other ways to deal with her problem. Even though she loved teaching, public speaking was such an obstacle that she considered changing careers.

   After she developed the basic skills of concentration practice, her therapist introduced her to loving-kindness and self-compassion. As she began to get curious about her fears, she realized she was terrified of being judged and found inadequate. Her father, a brilliant, tyrannical, and unstable man, had been critical of her throughout her childhood—whatever she did was not good enough, any achievement was derided and minimized. Carmen had assumed that her audience was a harsh and critical father, ridiculing and devaluing her every word.

   Carmen's therapist encouraged her to begin to experiment with shifting her internal beliefs about her audience. Before she began a lecture, she visualized sending everyone in her class warmth, loving-kindness, and compassion—*May you be safe. May you be healthy. May you be peaceful. May you live with ease.* As she practiced these phrases before each lecture, it helped her understand that her fears were rooted in her relationship with her father and that they were just thoughts, not necessarily truths. She began to see her class more clearly—some students were paying attention, some were texting, some were on their laptops (taking notes she hoped), while others were catching up on sleep. She let them be and realized that she could deliver her lecture without taking it all so personally.

   As the semester progressed and she got to know her students, her anxiety decreased. They were just kids doing the best they could, exhausted and overwhelmed with their lives just as she was with hers. Carmen decided that she didn't have to be an award-winning lecturer. She would notice her anxiety rising at the beginning of each lecture, but by sending loving-kindness and compassion to her audience it usually subsided in a few minutes. By the end of the school year she was able to teach without vomiting and panic attacks.

WORKING WITH EXTREME SUFFERING

The next practice is a variation of a meditation taught by many teachers, including Jack Kornfield (2008) and Paul Gilbert (2009a). It is particularly useful when patients have difficulty sending loving-kindness to themselves.

COMPASSIONATE BEING

- Start by sitting comfortably, finding your seat, and letting yourself settle.
- Take a few minutes to come into the present moment, anchoring with the breath, sounds, or touch points.
- Visualize a safe and serene place—a mountain, the beach, or a beautiful garden. Let this place be a refuge and a sanctuary for you. Let yourself rest here.
- Visualize a wise and compassionate being in front of you. This can be a favorite teacher, friend, or family member. It can also be a spiritual figure—perhaps the Buddha, Moses, Jesus Christ, Mohammed, or Kwan Yin, the goddess of compassion. It can even be a pet or other animal or a place in nature.
- Become aware of any pain or suffering that you are holding. Imagine what this being would say or do. What words would he or she offer? How would he or she comfort you? Listen deeply and see what arises. Allow yourself to receive the compassion and wisdom of this being.
- If your mind wanders, bring yourself back to this peaceful place and this compassionate being. Feel that you can take in some of his or her compassion and kindness.
- Let this place become an inner resource for you. Know that you can return here whenever you need support or sustenance.

Available in audio at *www.sittingtogether.com.*

CLINICAL ILLUSTRATION: WORKING WITH WHAT WE CAN'T CONTROL

Ian entered therapy to deal with the suicide of his brother, who had battled mental illness and addiction most of his life. He had tried to help his brother as much as he could, but had found his brother's demands overwhelming and irritating, especially once Ian had a wife and new baby.

What haunted him most was that his brother had called a few hours before he took his life. The baby was crying, Ian was sleep deprived, and he just didn't have the energy to deal with his brother. Ian told him he would call back. Now it was too late. He couldn't forgive himself for not talking to him that night. He wondered, over and over, if he could have saved him.

While Ian had taken a class on meditation, he was so consumed with guilt and regret that he couldn't sit still. At the beginning of treatment, he was unable to send compassion to himself. He felt he had abandoned his brother in his time of need. Ian blamed himself for not intervening, for not noticing his brother's desperation that night.

Even though it was clear that Ian could benefit from self-compassion, his therapist realized he wasn't ready to start there. So instead he introduced the practice of *Touch Points* (see Chapter 4, page 70) and *Labeling Emotions* (see Chapter 5, page 94) for a number of months. Using the phrases *May I be with this grief, May I make space for it* helped Ian feel grounded and stay with his feelings. At times he just noted, *This is what grief is like.*

Only after Ian had developed some acceptance of the suicide did his therapist moved on to the *Compassionate Being* meditation. Ian had grown up in a religious family and felt a connection with the Virgin Mary. He visualized the Virgin in front of him, sending love and understanding. As he worked with this practice daily, he felt that she was one being who could comprehend his suffering. Over many months of therapy, grief work, and meditation practice, his guilt began to let up. He had loved his brother and had done so much for him over many decades. It was tragic that he didn't talk to him that night, but he had no way of knowing that things were so dire—his brother had appeared to be doing better.

To help with the intense pain during the day, his therapist also introduced an informal practice from the MSC program called "Soften, Soothe, and Allow" (Germer, 2009; Neff, 2011). Ian would allow his body to soften, unclenching his teeth, relaxing the fists that he unconsciously was making, and breathing into the knot in his stomach. He would then put a hand on his heart, acknowledging his pain. He would say to himself: *My brother is gone. Let me accept this. May he rest in peace. May he be free of suffering.*

At the 1-year anniversary of his brother's death, Ian's sadness was still intense, but he realized that he wasn't responsible for his brother's illness, addiction, or death. Although Ian was never one to read poetry, a friend gave him a copy of these lines from a Pablo Neruda poem, which brought him some peace:

Perhaps the earth can teach us
as when everything seems dead
and later proves to be alive.*

To mark the anniversary, Ian started to work at a community suicide hotline, realizing that even though he hadn't saved his brother, at least he could learn to help others who were in despair.

As Germer (2009) points out, compassion is more than acceptance of what is happening to us in the moment. It is "acceptance of ourselves while we're in pain. . . . It's full acceptance: of the person, of the pain, and of our own reaction to the pain" (p. 33). When we cultivate compassion, we cultivate the ability to work with and open to deep levels of sorrow.

Other People

Sometimes our greatest emotional challenge involves other people. We've all been consumed, at one time or another, by interpersonal conflicts. The following practice can be useful when feeling stuck in negative feelings toward another person. Once some loving-kindness for oneself has been established, this practice can help transform our relationships with the challenging people in our lives. It is wise to start with someone who is mildly difficult and then move on to people we find to be more challenging. It can be used with friends, colleagues, a difficult boss, or family members. It can also shift a relationship with a difficult patient.

WORKING WITH A DIFFICULT PERSON

- Start by sitting comfortably, taking a few moments to ground yourself with sounds, touch points, or the breath.
- Begin practicing loving-kindness for yourself, using phrases such as *May I be safe. May I be healthy. May I be peaceful. May I live with ease.* Feel free to add additional or alternate phrases that speak to you.
- If it is hard to begin with yourself, start with a benefactor or

---

* Neruda, P. (1974). Keeping quiet. In *Extravagaira* (p. 26). (A. Reid, trans.). New York: Farrar, Straus & Giroux.

someone who has shown you kindness (as in the previous *Compassionate Being* exercise). Send the phrases of loving-kindness to this person and then, after a few minutes, fold yourself in, saying, *May we be safe, May we be healthy, May we be peaceful.* . . .

- Generate an image in your mind of someone who has been difficult for you. Don't start with the most challenging person in your life, but someone who is mildly to moderately difficult. Send loving-kindness to this person.

- If you feel overwhelmed or resistant, return to the breath or to the phrases for yourself. If you feel very upset, you can use the *Compassionate Being* practice as well.

- Take your time and feel free to stop after just a few minutes if the exercise becomes too difficult. Doing this practice for even 30 seconds can start to soften our feelings. Gradually increase the time as you are able. When you are ready, experiment with sending loving-kindness to someone who has been very challenging for you.

- End the practice by sending loving-kindness and compassion to yourself. See if you can carry this attitude into your next activity.

CLINICAL ILLUSTRATION: AN UNFORGIVABLE BETRAYAL

Alex had been married for over a decade when she discovered that her husband was having an affair. And to make matters worse, it was with someone she thought was a good friend. She was devastated and felt that the foundation of her life had been pulled out from under her.

In the divorce proceedings and custody battle, her husband was able to exploit her history of mental illness, arguing that she was not stable enough to be a good mother. She became panicked and fearful that she would lose custody of her son. In despair, she attempted suicide and needed yet another hospitalization. "I will never forgive him, ever," Alex declared.

She angrily confronted her ex-husband at their son's high school graduation. Many years later, her son announced his engagement. He told Alex that he wanted her at his wedding but she could not make a scene. Alex agreed to try. She had been working hard in therapy and had just started yoga as well. She approached the wedding as a challenge. She had not been able to establish a daily practice but when a friend told her she needed to meditate to get through the wedding she was motivated. "I need to be as together as possible," Alex said.

After learning to send loving-kindness and compassion to herself, a benefactor, a friend, a neutral person, and a moderately difficult boss, Alex was ready to work with her ex-husband. It had been nearly two decades since the divorce and Alex didn't want to take this resentment to her grave. When she started the practice, she was overwhelmed by memories, grief, and rage. At times it was too much for her. She returned to the practices of listening to sounds and sending loving-kindness to herself for what she had been through. When she couldn't sit, she would go for a leisurely walk, drink a cup of tea, call a friend, or play with her new puppy. At moments when the events all came flooding back, she comforted herself with the image of her benefactor sending her kindness and compassion.

With her therapist's help, Alex was able to acknowledge, for the first time, that her mental illness made her a difficult partner. While she couldn't forgive the betrayal and abandonment, she was able to soften a little. At least her ex-husband had been a reliable and devoted father. After months of preparation and practice, Alex anxiously anticipated the wedding. She splurged on a new dress so she would look as good as possible. With effort, saying her phrases during the ceremony, she was able to be cordial to her ex-husband and his wife, her ex-friend. Alex had never remarried, but asked a good friend to accompany her to the wedding for support. Attending the wedding and being courteous was a huge victory. "I will never condone my ex's behavior, but at least I was able to do the right thing for my son and his new wife."

Siegel and Germer (2012) write that compassion helps "cultivate a caring attitude toward ourselves and others, especially in the midst of suffering, which, in turn, allows us to hold our moment-to-moment experience with greater mindfulness and less resistance" (p. 11). This is just how it worked for Alex.

WHEN LIFE FEELS UNBEARABLE

Tonglen, the Tibetan Buddhist practice of giving and receiving, is designed to generate compassion and connect us with one another as a way to work with intense emotional pain (Chodron, 2001). The following version of the practice is adapted from the teaching of Lama Willa Miller (2009, 2012). It can help patients use intense physical or emotional pain as a vehicle for connection to others, transforming a symptom into an opportunity for growth.

CONNECTING WITH THE SUFFERING OF OTHERS

- Start by taking a few moments to allow yourself to settle. Use the anchor of the breath, sounds, or touch points to ground the attention and come into the present moment.

- Bring awareness to your experience of pain, either physical or emotional. Don't try to fix it or make it go away. See if you can lean into the experience. Notice what you are feeling. See if you can locate this feeling in the body.

- Pause for a moment and see if you can step back from the details of the story. If a strong feeling arises—anger, grief, sadness—note this with warmth and compassion.

- Take a few breaths and see if you can soften around the pain or suffering. See if there is any resistance in your body or mind. See if this, too, can soften. Try not to fight or struggle against it.

- Don't judge the experience or yourself. Allow yourself to have the full range of feelings, even if they are difficult to bear.

- Realize that you are not alone with these feelings or this experience. Know that there are many other people in the world with the same pain and the same suffering. Let this connect you with the other human beings who are feeling this way. Before this experience you could not have understood the suffering of these others. Now you can deepen your understanding.

- Allow compassion to arise, both for yourself and for all the other people who are in similar pain. Allow yourself to rest in this compassion. As the wish to ease suffering arises, say to yourself: *May all beings be free from suffering. May all beings know peace* (or similar phrases). Allow this to be an opening to a deeper connection with others.

- See if you can allow the separation between yourself and other suffering beings to begin to dissolve. Open to a state of oneness and spaciousness, letting things be as they are without trying to fix anything. Rest in the awareness of the present moment, letting thoughts and feelings arise and dissolve like clouds in an open sky.

• When you are ready, take a few deep breaths, stretch, wiggle fingers and toes, and open your eyes if they have been closed. See if you can carry a sense of the universality of pain into your encounters with others.

Available in audio at *www.sittingtogether.com*.

CLINICAL ILLUSTRATION: BEARING THE UNBEARABLE

Irina entered therapy after the tragic and senseless death of her only child. She had practiced mindfulness, but after her son's violent death she was unable to meditate, let alone eat, sleep, or work at her job. She had taken a medical leave to rest and try to heal. The loss was still fresh and she was in a state of shock. It was hard to believe that her son was really dead. She tried to make sense of his death but no meaning was possible. "Why me? What have I done to deserve this? Why is God punishing me?"

For the first 6 months of treatment, Irina screamed and wept—she called it "keening." Treatment focused on keeping her alive and as functional as possible. Some days she didn't think she would survive. She had no interest in mindfulness, she felt "too raw to go inside," but just wanted someone to be with her while she mourned.

In the beginning, it was impossible for her to sit with this enormous loss. As time passed, she began to talk about meditation, missing the comfort and grounding she once got from her practice, but wanted something "warmer" than concentration or open monitoring. We started with the *Connecting with the Suffering of Others* practice for a few minutes at first, then longer. During her intense mourning, this was the meditation that spoke to her—connecting with others who had lost a child was the only practice that made any sense.

As she continued to talk, grieve, and meditate in the years following her son's death, Irina began to see a new purpose in her life— she returned to school, studied for a degree in counseling, and began working with others who had lost a child in senseless acts of violence. She took comfort in the words of doctor and writer Rachel Naomi Remen that she found quoted in her local newspaper (Koven, 2012): "It is our wounds that enable us to be compassionate with the wounds of others" (p. 2).

Sharon Salzberg (1997) summarizes nicely the relationship among compassion, pain, and connection that Irina discovered:

Because compassion is a state of mind that is itself open, abundant, and inclusive, it allows us to meet pain more directly. With direct seeing, we know that we are not alone in our suffering, and that no one need feel alone when in pain. (p. 32)

THE INNER DARTH VADER

When people attempt the loving-kindness or compassion practices we've been describing, paradoxical responses often arise. Ambivalence is part of human nature—so when we try to make the mind do one thing, it often does the opposite.

There is a well-known story about the psychiatrist Milton Erickson. He was once on a horse farm. Someone was struggling to get a horse into a barn, but the harder the horse was pulled, the more he resisted. Erickson came up with a novel approach: *Pull the tail.* The horse bolted into his stall.

Many people find that when they try loving-kindness and compassion practices, negative judgments and unloving, unkind feelings arise, both toward themselves and others. It's important to remind ourselves and our patients that these feelings are all OK. The purpose of these exercises isn't just to generate loving and compassionate feelings so we can be more accepting of ourselves and others—helpful as this can be. Like concentration and other mindfulness practices, they're also designed to help illuminate how the mind operates and to help us more fully cultivate *awareness of current experience with acceptance.* So when we become aware of the inner Scrooge, Darth Vader, or other not-so-loving parts of our personality, the idea is to say "yes" to these. Loving-kindness and compassion practices can help us be aware and accepting of our darker side as well.

CHAPTER SEVEN

Equanimity Practice
Finding Balance

> True equanimity is not a withdrawal, it is a balanced
> opening to all aspects of life.
> —JOSEPH GOLDSTEIN and JACK KORNFIELD (1987, p. 201)

Equanimity is about finding balance in our lives. It is a steadiness of mind and a calm understanding that allows us to be with the constantly changing landscape of our world. While it is a capacity that is frequently explored in meditation centers, it is rarely discussed explicitly in psychological circles. For clinicians, however, equanimity can have immense value because it allows us to sit more comfortably with whatever comes up in our consulting rooms. It enables us to connect more deeply instead of spacing out or pushing anything away. It can help us not be overwhelmed by the pain we see, hear, and feel. In fact, burnout or "compassion fatigue," which can so readily befall therapists, may well be the result of empathy that is not tempered by equanimity and self-compassion (Siegel & Germer, 2012).

In difficult times, equanimity offers the promise that we can find perspective, no matter how extreme or difficult our circumstances. Equanimity develops as we learn to stay in the moment and keep our hearts open. It includes not only the capacity for emotional regulation but also for deep acceptance and undefended wisdom. No matter how painful or pleasant a situation might be, we learn to greet experience with balance and openness, to meet this moment fully "as a friend" (Boorstein, 2007, p. 124). When we are knocked off balance, we can return to center, accepting what life offers us with strength, flexibility, and humor. Sylvia Boorstein (2011b) finds inspiration for equanimity in her car's GPS system, noting that it never gets annoyed with her if she makes a mistake. So when she realizes that she has taken a wrong turn in relationships or clinical practice, rather than becoming angry she simply says, "Recalculating."

Like other aspects of acceptance, such as loving-kindness and compassion, equanimity can be cultivated. It is rooted in the insight and clear seeing developed through concentration and open monitoring practices. While sometimes misunderstood as indifference or the suppression of feeling, it actually involves being fully accepting of our emotions, responding with intelligence and wisdom instead of fear and confusion. Through equanimity we develop the courage to remain open to suffering. It is a steadiness without reactivity, without grasping, that helps us embrace rather than resist change. Equanimity is not passive, apathetic, or nihilistic, but is grounded in a broad perspective that sees the entire web of life. Considered to be one of the *brahmaviharas*, or limitless qualities of heart, in Buddhist psychology, it gives us the ability to meet life as it is and to come to, as meditation teacher Gina Sharpe (2011) says, "our best home."

As we saw in developing loving-kindness and compassion, to cultivate equanimity we can use phrases, repeated silently, to help us stay grounded when we lose our footing. Some of our favorites are:

All beings are on their own journey.
I care for you, but I can't control your happiness or unhappiness.
I may wish things to be otherwise, but may I accept this just as it is.
No matter how much I may wish otherwise, things are as they are.

As in other practices, we are not trying to force anything or to make ourselves or others experience any particular state of mind. The aim instead is to establish an intention to develop a particular attitude toward experience or quality of consciousness, to be with everything that arises and to hold it with patience and understanding.

An image often used to illustrate equanimity is that of a mountain.

No matter what the weather, the mountain remains steady and unwavering. As Goldstein and Kornfield (1987) write, "equanimity is the power of mind to experience the changes in the realm of form, the realm of feeling, the realm of mind, yet remain centered and unmoved" (p. 93).

The following meditation, which can be particularly effective in cultivating equanimity, was inspired by Jon Kabat-Zinn (1994). This practice is grounding and stabilizing. We find it helpful for patients weathering the storms of depression or anxiety, especially when they're going through a challenging transition, a significant loss, or an illness. As this practice doesn't depend on the cultivation of concentration or open monitoring, it can be used either in the beginning of treatment or later whenever balance or perspective is needed.

MOUNTAIN MEDITATION

- Start by sitting comfortably, taking a moment to ground and center yourself. Just be with the breath, sounds, touch points, or the loving-kindness phrases.

- Visualize a majestic mountain, either one that you have seen or one that you create with your imagination. It can be alone or part of a mountain range. This mountain changes, of course, like all things, but it changes slowly, in geologic time.

- Imagine your body becoming like the mountain—grounded, solid, still. Let the legs be the base, the arms and shoulders the slopes, the spine the axis, and the head the peak. Allow yourself to become centered, grounded, present.

- Visualize the mountain as the seasons begin to change. (You can begin in the current season and then slowly move through the others.) See it in autumn, surrounded by golden, warm light and brilliant colors. Gradually autumn gives way to winter, and the mountain is assaulted by intense and violent weather, by fog, snow, and ice. Notice how the mountain remains still, quiet, and steady through the storms.

- Watch as the seasons flow into each other. In spring, the snow melts, birds sing, and animals return. Wildflowers sprout and bloom. The mountain streams overflow with the melting snow.

- See the mountain in summer, bathed in light, quiet, solid, and majestic. Except for the highest peaks, the snow is gone. In every season clouds cover the mountain and then blow away, storms arise suddenly and pass.

- See the mountain through the course of a day, beginning with the rosy hues of dawn, then the clear light of morning, the deep golden light and shadows of afternoon. Watch as the day gives way to the rich colors of sunset and finally to the dark night sky, filled with stars and galaxies, endless space across the vast, clear heavens.

- See if you can sit like the mountain, still and grounded through the changes of weather, time, and seasons, allowing day and night to come and to go, accepting change, not resisting it.

- Take these qualities into your day, allowing the weather and seasons of life to come and go. Feel yourself being present, rooted, centered, and still, unmoved by storms, wind, cold, rain, heat, moments of darkness and light, joy and sorrow. Let life continue to unfold around you.

Available in audio at *www.sittingtogether.com*

As Kabat-Zinn (1994) suggests:

By becoming the mountain in our meditation, we can link up with its strength and stability, and adopt them for our own. We can use its energies to support our efforts to encounter each moment with mindfulness, equanimity and clarity . . . our emotional storms and crises, even the things that happen *to* us are much like the weather on the mountain. We tend to take it personally, but its strongest characteristic is impersonal . . . we come to know a deeper silence and stillness and wisdom than we may have thought possible, right within the storms. (p. 139)

For many people, the mountain meditation encourages a shift from identifying with the contents of the mind—the ever-changing kaleidoscope of thoughts, feelings, and images—to identifying with awareness itself. A related metaphor that can help develop this perspective involves imagining the mind to be like a vast sky. The contents of the sky are always changing, and at different times it might be filled with clouds, sun, rain, or snow, with daylight or the moon and stars. While its contents are variable, the sky itself is always there.

CLINICAL ILLUSTRATION: FIGHTING WITH THE GODS

Victoria, in woman in her 50s, entered therapy because she was feeling that her life was out of control. Barely over the death of her father,
she learned that the cancer she had battled earlier in life had returned.
In the past year, her husband had been diagnosed with early-onset
Alzheimer's disease, and their 17-year-old son was going through a
turbulent adolescence. Victoria wondered how she could endure treatment while caring for her husband and son and trying to work. "I just
want everything to go back to normal," she said.

As Victoria began to practice mindfulness, she worked with all the
different emotions that arose as she sat with the events of her life. First
she noticed grief over her father's death, her diagnosis, and her husband's
decline. She described it as being run over by a "Mack truck": "I don't
think I can handle all this sadness, it's too much, I don't think I can bear it,
I think I should stop therapy." Victoria's therapist helped her titrate these
emotions, opening to them one at a time so she wouldn't be overwhelmed.
At those times when she felt "run over" she would return to the sensations
of sitting and to the comfort of the sounds of the present moment.

As treatment continued, Victoria was gripped by intense fear about
her husband's deterioration, the loss of his support, and the uncertainty of
her own health and future. As she continued to practice, rage emerged,
"Why is this happening to me? I've been good. I've lived a moral life.
This makes no sense." She began to "fight with the gods" about her
fate. The intensity of her rage frightened her as she had never thought
of herself as an angry person. Her therapist suggested that she add the
question, "Can I make room for this anger?" In those times when she
couldn't, she changed the question to "Can I make room for this resistance?" Self-compassion practice also helped soothe her suffering.

Victoria requested a practice that would help her stay calm during
her medical procedures and that she could use when she "just couldn't
take it anymore." *Mountain Meditation* became a favorite—it helped her
feel that she could weather the storms of her life. For an informal practice when she wasn't able to sit and meditate, she used a practice taught
by meditation teacher Trudy Goodman (1999) of InsightLA, saying
to herself, *Body like mountain / breath like wind / mind and heart like sky.*
Victoria was someone who loved to hike and be outdoors; invoking
nature helped her keep a wider perspective.

YOU CAN'T STOP THE WAVES

In the 1970s, there was a famous poster of meditation teacher Swami
Satchidananda in flowing robes perfectly balanced on a surfboard

in rough seas. The caption was "You can't stop the waves, but you can learn to surf." The following is a practice of *urge surfing* (a term apparently coined by G. Alan Marlatt [Marlatt & Gordon, 1985; Marlatt, Bowen, & Lustyk, 2012]). It is a practice that is often used to work with addictions. We also teach this practice to help patients ride waves of strong emotion such as anger, sadness, or anxiety, as well as intense urges to eat, have sex, or act violently. When using this practice, it is important that the patient has the ability to concentrate as well as to stay with intense sensations. Before teaching it, also check that there is no history of trauma involving surfing, boating, or water skiing. One of us once taught this exercise to a group when a participant began to panic. It turned out that she had had a surfing accident decades ago, and the practice activated unintegrated memories of the event. If such an association arises, it can be helpful to shift to another metaphor such as riding a bicycle over hills or bumps or riding a roller coaster.

RIDING THE WAVE

- Start by sitting comfortably, taking a few moments to anchor using the touch points, breath, or loving-kindness phrases.

- Start by thinking about a recent situation in which you acted in a way that didn't serve you well—engaging in destructive behavior or substance abuse, yelling at someone, bingeing, or isolating yourself in reaction to a difficult situation or interaction.

- As you contemplate this scene, see if you can identify the feeling that immediately preceded the unskillful action. Stay with that feeling, and pause right before the wave of feeling "peaks." Try to stay balanced at that edge. Breathe and relax into the experience rather than fighting or resisting.

- As you observe this event, watch how the wave of feelings, thoughts, and sensations rises in intensity. See if you can stay with this "rising" rather than fighting the wave, or going under. See if you can ride the wave of your experience.

- Use your breath or the loving-kindness phrases as a surfboard to keep yourself steady. It's OK to "wobble" and to move back and forth as your try to find your balance. Just as in riding a real surfboard, constant subtle adjustment is necessary. See if you can find a dynamic rather than static balance.

- Stay as steady as you can until the wave begins to subside and fall. Return to your breath or touch points for a few moments before ending and returning to your day.

CLINICAL ILLUSTRATION: SNOW TIRES IN A STORM

Morgan had finished a tour of duty in Afghanistan, sustaining both inner and outer wounds. It had been hard to reintegrate into civilian life. Her family, especially her 3-year-old daughter, was delighted to have her back, but she was not the same. She was diagnosed with posttraumatic stress disorder and suffered from debilitating migraines, anxiety, and insomnia. She turned to alcohol to numb the pain. After she began drinking more and more, her addiction worsened until she was arrested for driving under the influence. It was in a detox center that she learned mindfulness practice. As she practiced coming back, again and again, to her experience in the present moment, she noticed that her flashbacks became less disturbing. Wanting to heal from her memories of combat and stay sober, Morgan also entered individual treatment and began attending Alcoholics Anonymous (AA).

Recovery was difficult and marked by frequent relapses. Morgan felt that she was a failure, a terrible mother, and a wretched human being. She worried that her life was ruined. When she relapsed, her therapist taught her to respond with compassion rather than self-injurious behavior. She worked with the phrases: *This is a difficult and painful time. I am not alone in my suffering. May I find balance. May I find wisdom.*

Her therapist then taught her the practice of *Riding the Wave*. At first this was difficult for her and she rejected the meditation. Her therapist did not force it. Morgan stayed with her compassion phrases, which she used when she needed them. However, after a binge that left her feeling shaken, she was willing to try again. "I need to get on top of this wave," she admitted, "or it's going to drown me." By learning to follow her urges, thoughtfully responding rather than automatically reacting, Morgan learned to ride out the difficult moments, knowing that they would pass. This helped her realize that a feeling doesn't last forever. Before, when she was having a hard time, she thought that she was locked into a "living hell" that would never end. In her therapy and in AA, Morgan learned that no matter how much pain she was in there was always a choice.

As Morgan practiced "surfing" and then grounding in the present moment, she felt less in the grip of her addiction. "I was in a shopping mall the other day and I got turned around. Luckily, they have these maps that get you oriented with a little arrow that says 'You are here.'

So now, whenever I'm feeling lost I just say to myself, 'Morgan, you are here.'"

She decided to plant a garden with her daughter, just as her mother had done with her. She signed up for a plot in a local community garden and began to plant tomatoes, cucumbers, and flowers that were easy to grow. Instead of drinking at the end of the day, she went to the plot to plant, weed, and then to harvest. The garden became both a way to stay grounded and a metaphor for her life. "I know that I can't erase all that has happened, but I can make good choices for me and my daughter. I can plant new seeds."

FINDING A STILL PLACE

We have adapted the next practice from a meditation taught by the Dalai Lama at Harvard University in 2003. It uses the metaphor of stillness beneath the waves to cultivate equanimity. This is a practice for turbulent times, such as job loss, illness, death, or trauma. We have found it to be effective when working with anxiety and depressive disorders. Like the *Mountain Meditation*, it can be used with patients who are relatively new to meditation (the Dalai Lama taught it to thousands of people, including many who had never meditated before). However, it is even more effective combined with the skill of concentration.

Since this practice can rekindle fears of water, it's a good idea to first check with your patient to make sure that the image of going under water is not disturbing.

ANCHOR AT THE BOTTOM OF A STORMY SEA

- Start by sitting comfortably, taking a few breaths to ground and center, using the practices of sound, touch points, the breath, or loving-kindness phrases.
- Visualize a boat anchored in a deep harbor. It is a tranquil, sunny day, and the water is still. But then the wind shifts suddenly. Dark clouds roll in, and the wind and waves start to batter the boat.
- Watch as the storm intensifies, bringing high winds, driving rain, hail, and enormous waves.
- Now imagine that you can drop below the waves, perhaps in a diving bell or in scuba gear, and bring your attention to the boat's anchor at the bottom of the ocean. Allow yourself to

rest here, seeing the storm and wind and waves high above you.

- Even though the storm is raging, see if you can find some spaciousness and stillness at the bottom of the ocean.
- Allow yourself to rest here, finding a quiet, still point in the midst of the storm.
- When you are ready, take a few deep breaths, stretch, and slowly open your eyes. As you return to the stormy surface, remember that you can return to the stillness whenever you need to.

Available in audio at *www.sittingtogether.com.*

CLINICAL ILLUSTRATION: WHEN THE THERAPIST NEEDS EQUANIMITY

Julia was a young therapist who had been working with George for several years. George had a history of impulsive behavior, suicide attempts, and numerous hospitalizations. He had recently become depressed after losing his job and was concerned about how he would pay the rent and survive. He had few friends and no family to help. Julia was concerned about him, but he assured her that he was fine and that he wouldn't hurt himself. She believed him.

The next day, when Julia retrieved her messages, she received one from George who had called in the middle of the night. He told her that he had nothing to live for, was taking stockpiled pills with alcohol, and would be dead by the time she received his message. Julia sprang into action and had George rushed to the hospital. At the intensive care unit, with George hovering between life and death, there was nothing more that she could do.

Julia began to berate herself and doubt her decisions—"How could I have missed this? Why did I believe him when he said he was fine? Why didn't I have a safety plan in place?" Her mind began to race—"What if he dies? I could get sued. I could lose my license. I would be disgraced. My career would be ruined. How will I survive?"

To help her stay in the moment and deal with her own catastrophic thinking, Julia first turned to the *Anchor at the Bottom of a Stormy Sea* meditation. Then she practiced a phrase that she learned in a mediation class: *Just this moment, nothing more, just this breath, right here, right now.* As she brought herself back, she realized that George wasn't dead yet. To help her find some balance, she turned to an equanimity phrase that had helped her before in difficult times: *As much as I would like things to be otherwise, things are as they are.* She also drew on another equanimity practice, saying, *George, I care about you. And you are on your own journey. Even though I may try, I cannot keep you from distress. I cannot make your decisions for you.*

George lived. He, too, had been frightened by his suicide attempt and was moved by Julia's efforts on his behalf. Julia, in turn, felt more connected to him and his distress. She sought out ongoing consultation for herself and connected George with a weekly psychotherapy group so he could get more support and she wouldn't be his only source of help.

The work of a therapist is never easy, especially when we take on high-risk patients. Freud (1937) spoke of the field as an "impossible profession," akin to child rearing and the governing of nations. As discussed in Chapter 1, we are wise to start with the best clinical training available. We then try to establish the moorings of good treatment: taking a careful history, developing an appropriate treatment plan and risk assessment, creating necessary documentation, and seeking consultation from experienced colleagues. While there are inevitable challenges in working as a psychotherapist, having the structure of regular consultation, along with adjunctive support such as group therapy or medications for our patients, can make it easier to have equanimity when caring for those who are most vulnerable.

TURNING TOWARD THE PAIN

Another way to help cultivate equanimity is by practicing feeling joy for others. This is an acceptance practice that is particularly useful when we are caught by envy and jealousy. We have used it with patients who are experiencing conflicts in relationships or a lot of negative judgments toward others. However, this is not a beginning practice. It works best when someone is grounded first in concentration, open monitoring, and compassion.

SYMPATHETIC JOY

- Sit comfortably, taking a few moments to ground and anchor. To help yourself settle, start with attending to sound, touch points, or the breath.
- As this practice can stir up strong feelings, spend a few minutes with the *Compassionate Body Scan* or loving-kindness phrases (see Chapter 6, page 105.)

- Bring your attention to the comparisons you make in your life, noticing when you think someone is smarter, more attractive, more fortunate, or more successful than you. Don't berate or judge yourself, just notice this.

- Choose a person, perhaps starting with someone who doesn't stir up strong emotions, and think of a source of joy in his or her life. See if you can appreciate this person's happiness. Silently repeat the phrases: *May your happiness and good fortune not leave you. May your happiness not diminish. May your good fortune continue.*

- When you are ready, try appreciating the happiness of a neutral person. Then, when you feel motivated, move on to the happiness of a difficult or challenging person.

- If this is difficult, or makes you feel off balance, return to loving-kindness phrases directed toward yourself. If it is really difficult, perhaps turn to the *Compassionate Being* practice (see Chapter 6, page 112). Expect this to be a process and don't worry if it is difficult. Even a few moments of practice can help you find more balance.

- See if you can carry this wishing of happiness for others into your next interpersonal interaction.

CLINICAL ILLUSTRATION: FINDING ANOTHER WAY

It had been a hard decade for Paulette. After struggling with infertility for years, she had finally conceived, only to miscarry at the end of her first trimester. Paulette's hormonal mood swings during fertility treatment and her subsequent profound depression and grief after the miscarriage were more than her husband had bargained for, and he eventually left the marriage to find someone who was "easier" and more "fun." In therapy she had been working on mourning and accepting her loss.

In the midst of her despair, Paulette received an invitation to her cousin's baby shower. They had a close but competitive relationship. Both Paulette's mother and aunt were pressuring her to "put her issues aside" and be there for her cousin. Paulette didn't want to go, but knew that if she didn't her cousin would be deeply offended and wouldn't speak to her. "What about me? Don't they care about how I feel?" she asked in therapy. There was a history of family rifts in previous generations and Paulette, a social worker, didn't want to create another cycle of ill will, anger, and resentment.

With her therapist's support, Paulette began to look at the pain of feeling invisible in her family of origin. To make this experience easier, her therapist also suggested she begin practicing compassion for herself. As a result, with a renewed sense of courage and self-acceptance, Paulette agreed to attend the shower, but she still worried she would break down during the event. In therapy, she was open to trying the practice of *Sympathetic Joy* to help her find some steadiness. She started practicing for a benefactor, a good friend, a neutral person, and then finally her cousin—her "challenging" person. On the day of the shower, her sister went with her. Realizing that seeing cute baby clothes was more than she could bear, Paulette gave herself permission to leave before her cousin opened the presents. She was helped by a phrase she learned from a meditation class: *Be there just enough.*

Seeing her cousin radiant and pregnant was extremely painful, but Paulette was able to see that her cousin had had no hand in her own infertility or the demise of her marriage. Paulette's family, even with their idiosyncrasies, was important to her, and she did not want to perpetuate the legacy of rivalry and competition in future generations.

Sharon Salzberg (2011) describes how this practice helps us see that life doesn't have to be a zero-sum game like tennis, in which your loss is my gain:

> Cultivating sympathetic joy opens the door to realizing that the happiness of others doesn't take anything away from us. In fact, the more joy and success there is in the world, the better it is for everyone. (p. 149)

RETHINKING FORGIVENESS

"Forgiveness means giving up all hope for a better past" (Kornfield, 2008, p. 346). We often think that forgiveness is about condoning an unforgivable or reprehensible act or ignoring injustice. But another way to see it is as creating space for a life free from the wounds of the past. We do not force ourselves to forget or deny that we have been hurt or abused. Instead, we try to come into a different relationship with our unresolved outrage or our guilt. In a very real sense, we do this practice out of compassion for ourselves. The Dalai Lama said,

> If you have an enemy and you think about them all the time—their faults and what they've done, and your grievances—then you don't

really enjoy anything. You can't eat; you can't get a good night's sleep. Why give them that satisfaction? (quoted in Salzberg, 2011, p. 171)

Through practicing forgiveness we learn to let go and start again. This is not a beginning practice. Introducing it prematurely could be experienced by a patient as an empathic failure or could result in the kind of "spiritual bypass" discussed in Chapter 1. So if a patient isn't ready, there's no need to push it. Let it come naturally. In cases of severe abuse, this practice may come only at the end of treatment or maybe not at all. It is best motivated by the patient's wishes, not the therapist's. If a patient is experiencing a lot of rage, it is generally best to work with the anger first, establishing some perspective. For those with intense self-loathing, it is good to start with forgiveness for oneself.

This practice is usually done in three parts: forgiveness for people you have harmed, forgiveness for the ways you have harmed yourself and, finally, forgiveness for those who have harmed you.

FORGIVENESS: LETTING GO OF POISON

- Start by sitting comfortably, taking a few breaths to come into the present. Ground and anchor yourself with the practice of sounds, the breath, or loving-kindness phrases.

- If at any point the practice gets too intense, feel free to return to your anchor.

- Start with the phrase *To anyone I have hurt or harmed, knowingly or unknowingly, I ask for forgiveness.* As images arise of people and events, say silently, *I ask your forgiveness.*

- Now consider the ways you have harmed and neglected yourself, and see if you can let go of any anger toward yourself for these actions or behaviors. *For all the ways I have harmed myself, knowingly or unknowingly, I offer forgiveness.*

- When you are ready (and don't rush or force this; it's OK to stay with the earlier steps for as long as you need), offer forgiveness to those who have harmed you. Don't expect immediate changes or healing. Think of this practice as setting an intention or planting some seeds. *To those who have hurt or harmed me, knowingly or unknowingly, I offer forgiveness.* If you're not yet ready to offer forgiveness, try substituting the following: *I willingly undertake the process of forgiveness.*

And if even that feels like too much—if rage, grief, or
sorrow arise and are overwhelming—just return to the
anchor.

- Take a few deep breaths, stretch, open your eyes. See if you
can maintain an attitude of forgiveness as you move through
your day.

CLINICAL ILLUSTRATION: "I WILL NEVER FORGIVE HER"

Heather first entered therapy in her early 30s to work on feeling stuck
with men, her career, and her living situation. It was a short-term treatment that helped her jump-start her life. There were issues she did not
want to address, especially her rage toward her mother, who had many
affairs and didn't protect Heather from being sexually abused by one of
her lovers. "I will never forgive her, ever." When her therapist tried to
get her to work on forgiveness, Heather pushed back and told him that
he wasn't listening to her. "I said NEVER, get it?" she fumed. Heather
terminated therapy shortly thereafter.

Fifteen years later, Heather returned to treatment. Her mother,
a breast cancer survivor, had had a recurrence of the disease and was
in hospice care. Heather had recently undergone surgery for her own
cancer. "I still hate her with a passion," Heather said, "but she doesn't
have much longer to live." Heather was ready to turn toward "the sharp
points."

She had studied meditation when she was younger, even traveling
to India and Thailand, in part to get away from her mother. Forgiveness was a practice she had ridiculed as not for her. "Maybe in another
life," she said wryly. "I want justice. She deserves to suffer. She ruined
my life." Heather was aware that her buried rage lived on somatically
in her chronic back pain and emotionally in her distrust of friends and
coworkers.

As Heather wasn't ready to work on forgiveness for her mother, her
therapist suggested she start with compassion for herself, then gradually
move toward compassion for a somewhat difficult person, and finally
for her mother. After several weeks, Heather slowly began to soften,
recognizing that her mother had no education or skills and that her
looks were her only commodity and source of power. She began to
understand her mother's desperate and destructive behavior.

As Heather softened, her therapist guided her to try asking for
forgiveness from those she had hurt—past boyfriends, her sisters, and
other friends and family members. She also looked at how she had

hurt herself through years of disordered eating and extreme exercise. Heather hadn't realized how hard she had been on her body and how rigid and controlling she had been with her friends.

For Heather, her mother's impending death finally motivated her to try forgiveness, hoping it would help release her from the toxic rage she had carried most of her life. Although her mother wasn't able to apologize for the neglect and abuse, Heather felt she had done her work and was certain she didn't want to hold on to her anger when her mother was in the grave. "My mother will always be a complicated figure for me, but there is no point in holding on to my hatred. She was horrible at times, but there were sweet, funny moments too. And she did give me life."

WHEN ONLY INDUSTRIAL STRENGTH WILL DO

The following practice is inspired by the teaching of Joanna Macy (2012). For some, it may involve a willing suspension of disbelief. But for those who can embrace it, this practice can offer a powerful shift in perspective. We have used it with patients whose lives have fallen apart because of the end of a marriage, the loss of a child or other loved one, the loss of a job, a shameful disgrace, or a life-threatening illness or accident. It is especially useful for those who are struggling to find some redeeming value in their suffering. While it is a good practice for extreme situations, we have also used it as a way to offer perspective on everyday disappointments. Before attempting this practice, it's best for the patient to have a firm grounding in concentration, open monitoring, and loving-kindness and compassion practices.

ACCEPTING THE CHALLENGE

- Start by sitting comfortably, taking a few minutes to ground and anchor, using the touch points, sounds, breath, or the loving-kindness phrases.

- Focus on a difficult circumstance in which you find yourself. Stay in touch with your thoughts, emotions, and fears. Notice what you feel in your body. Allow yourself to sit in the middle of all of it.

- Imagine, if you can, that before you were born you decided to have this experience to help you learn and to grow.

- Visualize that you are sitting with wise and compassionate elders who love and care for you. Discuss with them how these challenging events will help you develop new skills. What will you learn? Can you say "yes" to the events? See what this "silver lining" can teach you.

• Sit with your answers to these questions, seeing this difficulty with new eyes. See what happens if you imagine that you chose this situation rather than had it imposed on you.

• Imagine that you can embrace these circumstances as an opportunity to develop new skills and new strengths.

• As challenges arise during the rest of the day, consider how each might be an opportunity for growth.

CLINICAL ILLUSTRATION: "I CAN'T BELIEVE I LOST IT ALL."

Eduardo, a man in his early 60s, had been a successful businessman. He started his own company as a young man many years ago. He had worked long nights, weekends, holidays, and during vacations to help the business grow and flourish. But an economic downturn changed everything, and he was forced to file for bankruptcy. With no income, he also lost his house to foreclosure. Eduardo became deeply depressed. Just when he thought he had hit bottom, his second wife filed for divorce, saying that all his love had gone into the company and the marriage was bankrupt as well. Since the business had been his entire life, he had few friends or hobbies. He felt he was drowning. The final straw came when his mother, his greatest supporter and ally, was diagnosed with pancreatic cancer. "All this work, all this struggle, and what is left? It is gone, all gone," Eduardo lamented.

Eduardo's internist started him on an antidepressant, which helped him function. Eduardo was a fighter and wanted to start over, feeling that he still had a lot of life in him. He enrolled in a class at a local meditation center called Living with Uncertainty in Difficult Times and found it helpful. He then enrolled in more classes to help with his mounting anxiety. He started therapy as well to sort out what had gone wrong and to explore how to move ahead. Eduardo asked for an "industrial strength" practice to help him get through this time of great transition.

His therapist introduced Eduardo to the *Mountain Meditation*, which helped him get a footing. But he wanted more. "I need to see this differently," he said, "I want to turn this upside down and inside out." So his therapist taught him the practice of *Accepting the Challenge*. Eduardo imagined himself in front of a group of expert consultants whom he had hired to help him reorganize his life. As he worked with this practice, he realized that his business had become a pair of handcuffs. "It made me money," he said, "but it didn't help anyone, and now it's all gone. This is a chance for me to live a new life and maybe do some good."

THE MOST WONDROUS THING

In the great Indian epic the *Mahabharatha*, a wise king is asked to name the most remarkable thing in the world. He responded, "The most wondrous thing in the entire universe is that all around us people are dying and we don't believe that it will happen to us" (Salzberg, 2011, p. 23). No matter how hard we try, we cannot keep our bodies from aging and passing away. They will follow the laws of nature. This exercise can help us come to grips with existential reality. We use this practice with patients facing loss—of a marriage, a child, a parent, partner, friend, or even their own terminal illness. While this practice can be done as a visualization, it can also be done walking outside.

ALL THINGS MUST PASS

- Start by sitting comfortably, eyes open or closed, finding a posture of dignity. Spend a few moments grounding and centering with the touch points, breath, sound, or the loving-kindness phrases.
- Imagine a beautiful garden filled with your favorite flowers—all shapes, colors, and sizes. This garden can be one that you remember, one that you imagine, or one that you know currently.
- Let yourself walk among the flowers, noticing the colors, light, and fragrance. Notice that all flowers are in different phases of life—some are just budding, some are in full bloom, others are fading, and others have died. Bring equal attention to all—the beautiful full blooms as well as the dead flowers and leaves, even those that have been eaten by insects, revealing only their skeletal forms.
- Notice how even in the garden, everything has a beginning, a middle, and an end. Reflect on this fact in your life: all activities, all relationships, all endeavors arise and pass away.
- If you like, focus in on one particular flower. Notice the

light on the petals, the texture, the fragrance. Watch as
bees and butterflies come to drink its nectar. Know that
tomorrow, or the next day, this flower will wilt and fade.

- Let yourself rest in the garden, appreciating the beauty, the
preciousness, and the transience of it all, knowing that this is
the nature of life.

- Take a few breaths, stretch, and return to your day. See if
you can carry the awareness of impermanence into your next
activity.

CLINICAL ILLUSTRATION: LETTING GO

Lily entered therapy in her 70s. She had been diagnosed with cancer in
her 30s and had had several recurrences over the decades. Now she was
terminal. Her doctors couldn't believe that she was still alive. In spite
of her fragile health, Lily was still beautiful and had a contagious *joie
de vivre*. As a young woman she had been an actress and now was full
of stories about the theater, her travels, her lovers, and her "wild and
crazy" adventures. Children, and then cancer, had ended her career,
but she turned to painting and gardening as creative outlets in midlife.
She gained some artistic recognition and spoke proudly about having a
watercolor painting in a local show.

Lily wasn't ready to die. She didn't want to leave her husband, who
had recently had a heart attack. She worried about a daughter who suffered from bipolar illness. Lily had helped raise her 7-year-old grand-
daughter and would often care for her when her daughter was too ill to
parent. "I can't leave them," she said, "but I am so tired. Some days I
can barely get out of bed, especially after the chemo."

She was new to meditation but found it useful. Concentration
practices helped with the discomfort of medical procedures. She practiced *Labeling Emotions* (see Chapter 5, page 94) when she was in pain,
and self-compassion when she couldn't sleep because of worry. The
phrase "*My sweet body, you are doing the best you can*" helped her accept
that her body was failing. When she had trouble focusing because of
"chemo brain," she relied on an informal practice taught by psychologist Jan Surrey that involves coordinating some simple phrases with the
breath: "Breathing in, letting in/Breathing out, letting go" (personal
communication, July 29, 2012).

It was only when she was able to get her daughter into a good,
supportive therapy that she could finally begin to let go. "I don't want
to let go," she winked, "so I think of it as not holding on so tightly."

At this stage, the meditation practice that gave her most peace was one adapted from an ancient practice, in which yogis meditate on the decay and death of the body, often practicing among corpses in "charnel grounds" (R. D. Siegel, 2010, p. 304). As part of this contemplation, one reflects on what remains 100 years after death. While these are disturbing images, they are considered to be "strong medicine" that can put our lives in perspective.

Eventually, Lily decided to stop her weekly chemo, realizing that she had lived a rich and full life and she was tired. Her family would be able to get along without her. Lily said, "I can follow the cycles of nature; that is the way things are. No one should live forever."

Salzberg (1995) writes that to have

> the radiant calm and unswayed balance of mind that we call equanimity is to be like the earth. All things are cast upon the earth: beautiful and ugly things, frightful and lovable things, common and extraordinary things. The earth receives it all and quietly sustains its own integrity. (p. 193)

The practice of equanimity allows us to cultivate a vision as deep as the earth and as vast as the sky. It gives us perspective and an appreciation for the complexity and preciousness of life. It allows us to live wisely in the universe and to come to "our best home."

CHAPTER EIGHT

Making Mindfulness Accessible

Meditation isn't only for certain talented or already serene
people. You don't have to be an ace at sitting still; you don't
have to wait until you're uncrazed and decaffeinated. . . .
You can start right now. If you can breathe, you can
meditate.
                                        —SHARON SALZBERG (2011, p. 14)

W̄e sit around a table in a cramped room in a church basement under harsh fluorescent lights. The men and women, pierced and
tattooed, are attentive and hopeful. All of them have struggled with
homelessness and addiction. They are now living in a shelter, trying
to lead productive lives without drugs or alcohol. Committed to their
recovery and looking for tools to help prevent relapse, they asked a case
worker to organize a class in mindfulness meditation.

How do we make mindfulness accessible to the widest possible
range of patients? What are some of the challenges that arise and how
can we respond to them skillfully? How do we teach meditation to
people who have trouble paying attention or who live chaotic lives? As
discussed earlier, there are many ways to introduce mindfulness and the
form it takes will depend on the needs and abilities of our patients. In
this chapter, we explore how to introduce practices to individuals and

groups, in inpatient and outpatient settings, who may at first glance seem like poor candidates to benefit from them. We'll see that it's not necessary to turn all patients into dedicated meditators and that practices can be modified and presented so that virtually anyone can use them to find balance, kindness, and fulfillment in his or her life.

HOW TO START

People seek out mindfulness for a variety of reasons. As the men and women in the shelter introduce themselves, they talk about feeling overwhelmed, lost, and worried. Many have battled depression and anxiety as well as homelessness and addiction. Some are survivors of physical and sexual abuse as well. No one in the group has had any experience with meditation, and several are predictably skeptical.

BEING PRESENT

THERAPIST: It's good to be with you tonight. Thanks for telling me a little about yourselves. As this is new for all of you, I will keep these exercises short and simple, just 3 to 5 minutes each. After each practice, we'll have a chance to talk about what came up for you. Please let me know if you have questions or problems. These meditations are not one size fits all and we can fine-tune them so they work for you. The first thing we'll do is a simple exercise called *Being Present*.

- Start by sitting as comfortably as possible. You can close your eyes or let them rest softly on a spot of the floor.

- Take a few moments just to pause, letting go of your day.

- When you are ready, see if you can find a posture of dignity. You may find yourself sitting up a little straighter, but relaxed, not rigid. Often, when things are difficult, we can lose sight of our essential dignity, our goodness, our intelligence. See if you can feel that in yourself.

- And now, just notice that you are sitting. That you are here in this room. Begin to listen to the sounds in the room. This is an easy and direct way to come into the present moment. Just listen. See if you can listen with your entire being.

- You don't have to do anything special or force anything. Just let yourself settle. Simply notice the sounds in the room. The tick of the clock, the hum of the heater. Let these sounds be the focus of your attention, what we call an anchor.

- If your mind wanders into regrets about the past, or worries about the future, no problem. This is what the mind does. Just come back to the sounds in the room, to being present.
- Don't criticize yourself or beat yourself up. And if you do, just start again. Just listen.
- Our minds are so busy, running around and bouncing off the walls like a new puppy. Just gently bring yourself back to the room and back to listening to the sounds.
- If you get distracted, no problem . . . just start again. You haven't done anything wrong . . . you haven't messed up . . . gently, kindly bring yourself back to the room.
- When you are ready, wiggle your fingers and toes, stretch, and open your eyes.

"What Was That Like for You?"

When asked for feedback, several members of the group were eager to share what this initial experience of mindfulness was like for them, and were quite articulate about it:

RAMON: I thought you were supposed to make your mind go blank when you meditate. But mine just wouldn't stop. Are you sure that's OK?

THERAPIST: Absolutely. Actually, noticing how the mind keeps wandering and thinking about this and that is an important first step. Were you able to bring it back to the sounds?

RAMON: Yeah . . .

THERAPIST: Then that's good practice!

CRYSTAL: When I heard the clock ticking, it just reminded me of all the stuff I have to do. But I stayed with it, and I feel better now, a little less harried.

SHAKIRA: I kept wondering, "Why I am doing this? Am I wasting my time?" But it was good to stop, even for a minute or two. I feel a little more peaceful now.

KAYLA: I was surprised at how tense I was. I realized I was making a fist and clenching my jaw. Wow, I had no idea!

Not surprisingly, some of the group members were quiet and seemed unimpressed. Anita looked at a poster on the wall and didn't say anything, and Charles awoke from a quick nap. Not everyone takes to a given mindfulness practice.

You Don't Need to Sit

Since people often have trouble sitting still for long periods of time, especially if they're new to mindfulness practice, it's usually a good idea to dispel the notion that meditation has to be done in any special posture.

STANDING MEDITATION

THERAPIST: Contrary to popular belief, you can practice mindfulness in any position: sitting, standing, walking, or lying down. Mindfulness isn't anything weird or exotic, it's simply awareness of the present moment with kindness. It's knowing what you are doing while you are doing it. Let's try this together. Everyone raise a hand and wiggle your fingers. Know that you are moving your fingers. It's that simple. (*The group laughs and waves to one another.*) Mindfulness is knowing what you are experiencing while you are experiencing it.

In your introductions, many of you said that you were feeling overwhelmed and wanted to be more focused and grounded in your lives. You wanted a little more traction, like snow tires in a storm. The next practice helps you feel more anchored. Let's all stand up and try this together.

- Stretch for a minute and then feel the soles of your feet. Just notice the sensations of your feet on the ground.
- If you want, you can stomp your feet and make a little noise.
- You can shift your body forward and back, then side to side. Let yourself feel rooted, solid, connected to the earth.
- See if you can find your balance and come into your center. Try to stay over your feet.
- Now take a few breaths, and know that you are standing. Let yourself experiment with it, play with it. Feel the soles of your feet.
- You don't have to do anything special, just keep bringing

your attention back to the sensations of your feet on the
ground. Let yourself feel grounded.

- If your mind wanders and you get distracted, no problem.
  Just bring your attention back.

- Some people like to feel the ground beneath them,
  supporting them, meeting them. Feel free to try that if you
  like. Let yourself be anchored, strong.

- If you start thinking about other things, you haven't done
  it wrong, you haven't failed, the mind just wanders. Not a
  problem.

- And if it feels comfortable, bring your attention to
  your entire body. Notice any places that are tight or
  uncomfortable, and invite those places to soften. Notice
  where you are relaxed. No need to force anything, just
  acknowledge it, without judgment, with kind attention. Let
  yourself be in your body for a few moments.

- When you are ready, wiggle your fingers and toes, stretch,
  and return to your seat.

"How Can You Find Your Center If You Never Had One?"

Once again, the therapist asks for comments. Checking in frequently
and asking for feedback is important, especially with beginners. The
group seems pleased that mindfulness isn't only about sitting still.

TOMAS: I liked being able to stomp my feet. I thought we were
going to be silent and everything. It helped me release some
tension and wake up a little.

CRYSTAL: I just liked feeling my feet on the ground.

THERAPIST: Great! Can anyone think of some ways you could use
this during the day?

CRYSTAL: Well, I just started a new job as a waitress and it's very
stressful, especially when the customers are rude. I could try
to feel the soles of my feet when I'm about to melt down!

THERAPIST: And it isn't that you suddenly won't melt down or
have hard times. But you can use this tool to help return to
center.

SHAKIRA: I could try it when I'm waiting for the bus, worried I'm
going to be late.

THERAPIST: One of the best things about these practices is that they're completely portable. You can do them anywhere.

CHARLES: This is a bunch of shit. How can you find a center if you never had one?

CRYSTAL: Hey, Charles, it's like what they tell us in our 12-step programs. It's in everyone.

THERAPIST: Charles, that's a really important question, a great question. Just remember, these are skills we all can learn. Like playing baseball or riding a bike. It takes practice, but everyone can learn. Even if we never got this in childhood. And many of us didn't.

CHARLES: (*Shrugs his shoulders and looks unconvinced.*)

Finding the Breath

As discussed in Chapter 1, bringing attention to the belly, chest, and neck, as in traditional meditations that use the breath as an object, can be problematic for many patients. And yet the breath is particularly handy as an object of attention, since it's always present. Here is a non-threatening way to introduce breath-focused practice that is less likely to bring up threatening thoughts or feelings.

FEELING THREE BREATHS

THERAPIST: A lot of meditation classes start by teaching you to focus on your breath. Some people find it to be a useful tool. If you have had asthma or other breathing problems, this may not be a good fit, however. Often people who are anxious, or have experienced trauma, also don't feel comfortable with it. But since this practice is only three breaths, it's a pretty safe experiment. If it doesn't work for you, just listen to sounds or feel the soles of your feet.

Remember, no matter where you are, or what is happening, you can always feel your breath. One of my meditation teachers, Trudy Goodman, taught that we could shift our state of mind with just three breaths. So let's try this and see what you notice.

- Sit comfortably, finding a posture of dignity. Just gather your attention. Know that you are here and that you are sitting.

- When you are ready, bring your attention to the breath. Let yourself get curious. What is it that lets you know that you are breathing? Sometimes it is the rise and fall of the chest, or the expansion of the belly, or the air at the nostrils. See where you notice the breath most strongly.

- Bring your attention to your inhalation, feeling the sensations as the air fills your body, and then feel the exhalation.

- You don't have to force it or control it. There is no way to do it wrong. Just find your natural breath.

- Notice the next inhalation, paying attention to all the sensations, and then feel the exhalation. You can put a hand on your belly to help you feel the breath.

- The breath is your companion. It has been with you since birth and will be there until you die. See if you can rest in the breath.

- Bring all your attention and awareness to feeling the third inhalation and exhalation. Let the breath be a friend.

- Allow yourself to rest there for a moment, being present with the breath. Let this be a resource, a refuge that you can return to whenever you need it.

- When you are ready, wiggle your fingers and toes, stretch, and open your eyes if they were closed.

"What Did You Notice?"

There will be a range of reactions to almost every practice, and no one practice will speak to every person.

CRYSTAL: I've had asthma my whole life. I hate thinking about my breath.

RAMON: I like this practice. I feel more peaceful, a little less distracted.

SHAKIRA: I like the idea that I could find my breath any time or any place.

TOMAS: I like the fact that this is so simple and that no one else needs to know I'm practicing mindfulness.

The therapist also taught the class a variation of a breathing practice from the Zen master Thich Nhat Hanh that they can use in daily life: "Breathing in, I know that I am breathing in; breathing out, I know that I am breathing out." The group tries this for a minute and then responds:

KAYLA: I like standing better.

CHARLES: I guess the breath is OK.

ANITA: I like relaxation better lying down.

All of these responses are fine. There is no right way to practice. Our aim as therapists is to help people feel more alive and more present and, if possible, to help them find a practice that resonates for them. This often involves a good deal of experimentation.

Adding Some Kindness

Many people who are reluctant to try meditation practice have minds that create a lot of negative judgments: toward themselves, toward others, and toward meditation practices. Some will respond well to simple practices that help relax this critical tendency.

OPENING TO KINDNESS

THERAPIST: The final practice that I would like to explore with you tonight is the practice of loving-kindness. There is an ancient saying that we could search all over the world and not find anyone more deserving of our love and compassion than ourselves. Sometimes we don't feel we deserve kindness and care. Often when things are difficult we think we need to be critical of ourselves to change, to motivate ourselves, but actually the opposite is true. We respond better to kindness than to criticism. This might seem hard to believe and certainly may not be the way you were raised. We often think that it is self-indulgent to be kind to ourselves. But it isn't. Compassion for ourselves can help us survive hard times.

- Start by sitting comfortably, eyes open or closed, finding a posture of dignity. Give yourself a few moments to settle.
- Allow yourself to ground or find your center with sounds, the soles of your feet, or your breath.
- Think of a person who has been kind to you. It could be

a grandparent, a teacher, a parent, a sibling, or a friend. It could even be a beloved pet, like a dog or a cat.

- Allow yourself to feel this kindness, this warmth. See if you can take it in. Imagine this person, this being, gazing at you with warmth and understanding, with kindness and compassion.
- Imagine that this person is wishing you well, sending you a blessing, and perhaps saying these words: *May you be safe and protected. May you be healthy. May you be held in kindness and compassion.*
- See if you can receive this care and kindness, take in that this person cares about you.
- Take a moment to see if there are other words that you might need to hear. Sometimes people in recovery like these phrases: *May you be kind to your body. May you learn to love and accept yourself. May you forgive yourself.*
- If you like, you can simplify the phrases, using them as a resource to help you steady. You can just say: *Safe. Protected. Healthy. Kind. Compassion. Forgiveness.*
- When you are ready, take a few breaths, wiggle your fingers and toes, stretch, and open your eyes.

"What Came Up for You?"

Loving-kindness practice often brings up strong reactions in people, and this group was no exception.

CRYSTAL: I'm trying to learn not to hate myself for all my mistakes. And boy, have I fucked up!

RAMON: I like the idea of forgiving myself and starting again. That's good.

SHAKIRA: Not many people have been kind to me, but it was good to think about the few who have been.

CHARLES: It didn't do much for me.

THERAPIST: Sometimes we *don't* feel much when we do this practice. Or sometimes we even feel sad or angry. And that's OK. When we practice loving-kindness, it's like planting seeds. We're expressing an intention to be kind to ourselves, even if we're not feeling it right now.

KAYLA: I like some of those phrases. But how can I remember
them when I need them?

THERAPIST: I have a handout with the phrases on it that I'll give
to all of you in just a few minutes when we end. Some people
actually write them down on little flash cards and carry them
around as a reminder. Like the other practices we've done
today, this practice of kindness is portable. You can do it waking up, walking, driving, on the bus, at work, with a difficult
person, during a confrontation. And use it in hard times. That
is often when you need it the most. You know, I teach a class
on self-compassion with a colleague. And one of the things
we say is "Why not give yourself the kindness and love you
deserve but can't count on getting from others during the day,
even those who love you." All of these exercises are skills that
you can learn. And they can make a huge difference in your
life.

So I see our time is up for today. Here are the handouts.
Thanks again for inviting me to talk with you. It's been a
pleasure. [See *www.sittingtogether.com* for reproducible handouts; see the Appendix, page 211, for examples of flash cards.]

"THERE'S A TORNADO IN ME"

As discussed in Chapter 1, it's wise to be careful when introducing
mindfulness practices to people with particularly fragile or vulnerable
personalities. But even people with severe psychiatric disorders, who
have great difficulty functioning in the world, can benefit from appropriate practices introduced thoughtfully. Consider, for example, one
of our experiences in introducing mindfulness practices to Ximena, a
woman hospitalized with major mental illness.

Ximena's son found his 60-year-old mother cowering under the
kitchen table, shaking and sobbing. She had stopped eating or caring
for herself. She was no stranger to the inpatient unit; her long history of
mental illness had required frequent hospitalizations. The past year had
been especially difficult. Her youngest daughter, who was pregnant,
had been killed in a gang-related shooting. After her death Ximena
had been unable to work. Most days she stayed in bed, rocking back

and forth and crying, "They killed my baby, they killed my baby." She had stopped taking her medication, fearing that it was poison. When admitted she was floridly psychotic, experiencing auditory and visual hallucinations.

Introducing mindfulness in an inpatient setting with psychotic or dissociative patients should always be done with care. One of us once tried what seemed like a simple grounding practice of bringing awareness to the hands with a patient who was high functioning and appeared to be stable. After 30 seconds of this she looked up quizzically and asked, "But how can I tell if these are my hands or my mother's?" Sometimes things aren't so simple.

Before introducing a practice, we usually frame it as an experiment that the patient can stop if it feels uncomfortable. Then, if a practice does go south, we try to minimize any blame or shame the patient might be feeling by pointing out that this doesn't mean the patient has "failed." It simply means that this particular practice is not a good fit at this time.

As an inpatient, Ximena received daily individual therapy. One morning she entered the office looking disheveled and frightened.

"There's a tornado in here," she said in a panicked voice.

"No, Ximena," her therapist said calmly, thinking she was supporting her reality testing. "There isn't a tornado here. You are in the hospital."

She looked her therapist in the eye and said, "There was a tornado in the area and it entered my body."

Her therapist quickly realized her error. She had missed Ximena's underlying meaning. She paused and took a few breaths. Her therapist realized that she was feeling anxious and upset, and didn't know how to help. She wanted to repair this breech.

"Yes," her therapist said, "there have been some mighty fierce winds recently. And some really bad storms. It must feel like you have been in the middle of that tornado."

Ximena felt understood and began to weep, quietly at first and then with deep, heaving sobs. Her therapist sat with her silently, not saying anything, not trying to fix it. She knew that what she could offer Ximena at that moment was her presence and her willingness to sit with her during her grief. Her own mindfulness practice helped her stay present.

During her stay at the hospital, Ximena went in and out of psychosis. One morning she came in distressed and told her therapist that wolves were attacking her, tearing her up from the inside. Her therapist said that it must be frightening, and hard to feel safe after what had happened to her.

Once again Ximena began to cry and said, "I feel like I'm being eaten alive." Her therapist sat with her quietly, just being present and sitting with her grief.

Introducing Awareness of the Body

With medication and the safety of the hospital, Ximena's hallucinations abated and she began to eat again. When she had stabilized and had developed a good treatment alliance, her therapist asked Ximena if they could try an exercise together that might be grounding and comforting. If she didn't like it, they could stop at any time. She agreed.

They stood up together and Ximena was asked just to feel the soles of her feet. Could she feel the floor underneath supporting her? She could.

"Do you feel present in your body, even just a little?" her therapist asked.

"I don't know," Ximena said. "What does that mean?"

"That's an excellent question. It can be hard to put into words. Let's try swinging our arms back and forth, up and down. Just a little at a time. See if you can feel the sensations. Just feel your arms. Now pause. Check in, is there any place in your body where you feel grounded and safe?"

Ximena nodded, "My feet."

It turned out that Ximena had been an athlete when she was young and loved to play soccer with her brothers.

"OK, let's work with that. Try kicking your feet, like you are about to kick a ball."

"Now I feel it," she said brightly.

It was the first time that her therapist had seen Ximena smile. "Stay with that for a minute, just feeling your feet," she suggested.

In subsequent sessions, Ximina and her therapist continued to talk about her daughter's death, but saved the last 10 minutes of the session for brief mindfulness exercises. They practiced awareness of body sensations to help Ximena return to the present moment, especially when she was triggered. In addition to practicing awareness of the arms and legs, they experimented with walking down the long corridors of the unit. "Just feel your feet as you walk, feeling the sensations. It's fine to feel just a little at a time. Just lightly touch those sensations. And you can swing your arms if you like."

While Ximena was not a candidate for sitting meditation or for closing her eyes and going inside, she enjoyed the modified walking meditation. As she worked with small bits of awareness at a time, she could tolerate and even enjoy the experience. This practice helped her stay in her body and the present moment for longer periods of time, increasing what Dan Siegel (2010) calls the "zone of tolerance." And in the moments when she felt that the wolves or the tornados were approaching again, she would remind herself, "Feel the soles of your feet. Just walk. Feel your arms. Feel your legs." As they worked with this exercise day after day, Ximena was able to achieve some increased stability and resilience, develop a capacity to soothe herself, and was able (on a good day) to return to the present moment when hijacked by a memory of past trauma. When she found herself "slipping away," Ximena learned to bring herself back by saying, "Here, let me be here." Two mindfulness phrases helped her stay in the present, rather than dwell in traumatic memories: *If it isn't happening now, it isn't happening;* and *That was then, this is now.*

"We Are Not Alone"

Another informal practice with which Ximena resonated was a simplified variation of *tonglen* (see Chapter 6, page 116, and the Appendix). In this version, she would think of all the mothers and families in her community who had lost children or loved ones to violence. She would acknowledge their loss, pause, and take a breath. As she breathed out, she would send kindness and understanding to these families and others around the world who had suffered terrible loss. And then she would whisper to herself, "We are not alone."

After several weeks, as she prepared to go home, Ximena was able to sum up what she had learned: "When you lose a child, it isn't something you ever get over. She was part of my body, my blood, my bones. It's your future too that's gone. I think of her every day. But I have other children. And they need me. Life goes on. I can't just stay in bed."

NOTHING WEIRD

As the examples so far indicate, many formal meditation practices can be adapted for people who do not want to practice meditation or seem initially like poor candidates. Practices can even be woven into the fabric of therapy so that they become part of an ongoing interaction. In the following case, one of us simplified a meditation taught by Joan Halifax (2008, pp. 14–17) and changed it into a dialogue that the patient could explore with her eyes open.

"I'll talk with you," Loretta warned as she sat down for her initial appointment, "but promise me, nothing weird, and I ain't closing my eyes."

Her therapist laughed and responded. "That's not a problem. We can do therapy with eyes open."

"Good," she responded, relaxing a little. "I was raised a devout Christian and I don't do any new age crap."

A straight-talking, no-nonsense divorced woman in her 50s, Loretta was sent by her internist, who suggested that meditation could help her manage her stress. She worked as a sales representative for a pharmaceutical company, a job that required frequent travel. Loretta had been experiencing heart palpitations and was using over-the-counter drugs to help with sleep. She was also battling obesity, which she claimed was a losing battle: "I like my alcohol, my sugar, and my comfort food." She also complained of chronic headaches and back pain, which she attributed to long hours in the car. "My doctor wanted me to try yoga, but there is no way I am putting on some spandex leotard," she said as slapped her thigh and laughed. "Can you imagine that?"

Outgoing, sociable, always smiling, Loretta loved to talk. She was a born storyteller with a wonderful sense of humor. Raised as an "army brat," she learned to make friends easily. "I got really good at fitting in and getting people to like me," she said with a radiant smile.

For the first few months of therapy, Loretta was happy to tell stories about her life and travels. She responded well to the structured interventions of cognitive-behavioral therapy. She started an exercise program to decrease her high blood pressure and cholesterol, and was making wiser food choices with the help of an online weight loss program.

One day, however, she came in with a disturbing dream that she couldn't shake. It was the first session where she wasn't smiling. In the dream, someone was trying to suffocate her with a pillow and she was trying to fight him off. She tried to scream for help but no one came.

"I don't know why I can't just let it go," she said. "It was just a silly old dream. I usually don't pay any attention to my dreams."

"An old dream," her therapist repeated. "So you've had that dream before?"

"Yeah, for years, but I can usually let it go. I don't know why it got under my skin this time."

Her therapist asked Loretta if she'd like to try a new way to work with it, and she somewhat reluctantly agreed.

Bringing Mindful Awareness to the Body

Loretta's therapist asked her to take a few breaths and become aware of her body. "It's fine to keep the eyes open. Just see what you notice, get curious about what you feel in your body."

Loretta looked skeptical, but began paying attention. After a few minutes she said, "I feel some pressure in my neck and throat."

"Can you stay with it?" her therapist asked.

Loretta nodded and her therapist continued. "Let me know if it gets overwhelming. Tell me what you are aware of."

After a few moments, Loretta's tone changed. "I haven't wanted to think about this. I've been running so fast and working so hard that I didn't have to. This is why I hate to go to sleep. I can't push it away then."

Then she took a deep breath and began to cry. "When I was about 10, we had just moved to a new home in Savannah. This older boy, who was 14 or so, lived in the neighborhood. He was nice looking, from a crazy family, but he reached out to me. We would just hang out together. My mother was distracted with the move and the younger kids. She was happy that I found a new friend so quickly. It all started innocently, just talking, spending time together. But one rainy day things got sexual. I wanted to please him, so I went along. I didn't fight. And it went on for months. I didn't want to lose him or make him angry. I thought he was my friend. He told me he would strangle me if I told anyone. So I didn't. I just started eating. There was a donut shop nearby and they had the best honey-glazed donuts in the world. I can still smell them now. That was my comfort food. I never breathed a word to anyone, not even my mother. She never asked why I gained 30 pounds. She just thought it was adolescence. And then we moved again. I've been carrying this secret for years."

Loretta continued to weep. "I was always scared of sex after that. Never liked it, because it made me feel dirty. And it ruined my marriage. My ex just found someone else who could satisfy him. And I started eating even more."

In the sessions that followed, Loretta didn't smile much. After a month of working with memories of the abuse, her headaches were less frequent. But sleeping was still difficult and she worried about having more bad dreams.

Eye-Opening Meditation

At this point, her therapist asked Loretta if she'd like to learn an exercise she could practice when she was trying to fall asleep.

"Sure," she said. "But you know me. Nothing weird."

"Don't worry," her therapist laughed, "we can do this as a dialogue."

Here's how the rest of the dialogue went:

DIALOGUE MEDITATION

THERAPIST: Begin by sitting comfortably, feeling your body on the chair and your feet on the floor. It's fine to keep your eyes open. See if you can feel the strength of your spine. If you like, you can move side to side, and front to back. Feel how your back is strong and flexible. You might even like to feel the vertebrae all stacked one on top of another. Notice how your back keeps you erect and upright. How it holds up. You can even say to yourself, "Strong back."

LORETTA: I like this. So much of the time I feel weak, not good enough. It's nice to feel strong for a change.

THERAPIST: Just stay with it. Let yourself really experience your strength.

LORETTA: People would always put me down. My father, my husband. Always finding fault with what I did, what I said, how I dressed. Even my cooking. Just couldn't win.

THERAPIST: Keep returning to what you feel in your body.

LORETTA: This reminds me of how I feel after my aerobics class. Someone you can't mess with, someone you can't push around.

THERAPIST: OK, now stay with that, allow yourself to feel that strong back.

LORETTA: I'm feeling it!

THERAPIST: And when you're ready, let's try balancing it out with a little softness, especially for those times when you feel tense or worried. If you like, put a hand on your belly and a hand on your heart. Just invite those muscles to soften. No need to force anything, just notice what you're feeling.

LORETTA: My stomach is always in knots. Really tight. And I'm always late, which only makes it worse.

THERAPIST: OK, good. See if you can get interested in what you notice. And if you like, continue to feel your belly soften. Just pause, giving it a few minutes. And when you're ready, move to your chest, your shoulders, your neck and throat. No rush, let your body unwind a little. Take it slow, just bring attention to these places in your body. And when you're ready, notice your jaw. Invite it to soften. Just spend a few minutes there.

LORETTA: Yikes! Sister, is that tight! My dentist even told me to do some stress reduction. I clench my jaw and grind my teeth so much I broke a tooth!

THERAPIST: Yes, we often store tension in the jaw. Now bring attention to your eyes, letting them soften and release. Make your gaze soft. Instead of looking at an object with a laserlike focus, let your eyes soften and your vision blur for a moment, letting in everything in the perceptual field. It's like using a wide-angle lens rather than zooming in on something. And if you like you can say to yourself, "Soft front."

LORETTA: I like this. My headaches often start with my eyes.

THERAPIST: See if you can stay with this for just another minute. Letting the front of the body soften and open, but still feeling the strength or your spine. Feel both of them together. And if you like, shift back and forth, feeling strong and feeling open. Holding both, finding some balance. And when you're ready, wiggle your fingers and toes, stretch, and let me know how that was for you.

LORETTA: This was good. And not too weird! You know, I need to be strong, but I also need to be open, especially with my customers and my friends and family.

By introducing Loretta to some simple mindfulness exercises in the form of a dialogue, she was able to not only confront some painful childhood memories but also begin to notice and change her relationship to the tension she had been holding in her body.

The practices in this chapter are "entry-level" exercises that can be done with virtually any patient at any point in treatment. We can also use them ourselves as clinicians when we're just beginning mindfulness practice or feeling particularly vulnerable or overwhelmed. As discussed earlier, deciding when and how to move on to more intensive practices, some of which are only appropriate for particular individuals at particular stages of therapy, involves clinical judgment, in-depth knowledge of our patients, and firsthand experience with the practices. It is often best to do this in stages, beginning with one type of practice and moving to others either as we or our patients develop requisite skills or in response to changing psychological states. In the next chapter, we provide examples of how to sequence practices throughout the course of treatment with a variety of different disorders.

CHAPTER NINE

The Art of Sequencing

> There is suffering, there is the cause of suffering, and there
> is the end of suffering. Wherever you are, is the place to
> realize these truths.
> —Ajahn Chah (in Kornfield, 2011, p. 250)

Finding the optimal combination of mindfulness practices to address the clinical needs of an individual patient at different points in treatment is more art than science. Clearly, one size does not fit all. What's more, there is no simple recipe or formula for choosing techniques. We need to rely on our clinical judgment combined with our understanding of how these practices affect the mind and heart. While therapists often worry that they don't know which practice might be best at a given moment, our most important contribution lies beyond choosing a technique—it is bringing our presence, intelligence, and care for the suffering of our patients into the consulting room. As the Zen master Rinzai suggested, "Concentrate on what you do, wholly, just here and now, and quite naturally you will find the way" (Cambridge Insight Meditation Center, 2012). Nonetheless, guidelines can be helpful, and this chapter offers examples of how mindfulness practices can be sequenced in psychotherapy.

Many meditation teachers present practices in a traditional sequence, starting with concentration, followed by open monitoring, then loving-kindness and compassion, and finally equanimity. As of yet, there is no empirical research supporting or challenging this or any other approach. We have only anecdotal data to guide us. What follows, therefore, are suggestions from the laboratory of the clinical hour. We encourage you to experiment, trying to discern what seems to work for you and your particular patients.

One way to conceptualize the interrelationship of various mindfulness practices is through the analogy of a house. Concentration is the foundation; it is hard to gain insights or stay present with difficult thoughts, images, and emotions without this basic skill. Open monitoring can be thought of as the structure of the house, providing a framework. When storms arise, it offers shelter and protection as we adopt an attitude that allows us to stay with a wider and wider variety of experiences. Loving-kindness and compassion are the hearth, providing warmth, comfort, and fostering good will among the inhabitants. Equanimity, like the windows, allows light and a wider perspective to enter, enabling us to see both inside and outside more clearly.

However eager we may be to introduce our patients to mindfulness practices, it is important to assess their needs first, taking a careful history, considering their strengths and vulnerabilities, and discerning whether a given practice is a good fit. Before rushing in to be helpful, even if we are confident of the potential benefits of mindfulness, we need to meet our patients where they are, not where we want them to be. One eager clinician spent her weekend at a mindfulness workshop and was excited to share all that she learned with a new patient on Monday morning. The patient, however, was not interested, in part because her mother had abandoned the family to "find herself" in an ashram in India. The therapist's interest in mindfulness was experienced as a sign that she was not the "right person." This first session was also the last.

Just as a real estate agent would not push a Victorian suburban home on a client who wants an urban high-rise, we need to attend to the needs and histories of our patients. Even with the pressures of accountability, it's important to take time first to listen and to form an alliance. Many patients won't be ready for anything beyond entry-level practices (see Chapter 8) until the middle or end of a treatment. As in any therapeutic relationship, in mindfulness-oriented psychotherapy, vulnerabilities, character issues, transference, and countertransference come into play. Reenactments and suicidal impulses don't cease just because we've incorporated mindfulness techniques into our therapy, nor will projection, idealization, and other defenses or coping strategies disappear.

WORKING WITH THINGS AS THEY ARE

There is a story that offers an alternative to trying too hard to "fix" our patients or have them embrace mindfulness. As the tale goes, when the British colonized India they missed being able to play golf, so they set about constructing golf courses. A problem arose, however, when the local monkeys joined in the game, creating havoc by throwing the little white balls wherever they liked. The frustrated golfers formed a committee to address the monkey problem. First they decided to build a high fence around the golf course, but the monkeys delighted in climbing over it. The committee then decided to round up the monkeys and cart them away. But the monkeys returned. After intense discussions, one of the golfers had an idea. "Let's play the ball where the monkey drops it."

This story is useful to remember when we find ourselves wanting things to be different than they are, including wanting a patient to do things our way—whether leaving an abusive relationship, stopping an addictive behavior, being less narcissistic or self-destructive, or taking up a particular sequence of mindfulness practices. We have to temper our enthusiasm and channel it into understanding our patients so we can offer them interventions, skills, insights, and practices from which they are ready and equipped to benefit.

CLINICAL ILLUSTRATION: ALREADY BROKEN

Holly was an articulate, intelligent, appealing young woman with enormous potential. Unfortunately, her chronic and severe depression made it difficult for her to sustain work or intimate relationships. While she periodically made friends, they soon became exhausted by her demands and she found herself alone and bereft.

Her young, enthusiastic therapist tried every technique she could find to "cure" Holly's depression. Holly tried psychodynamic therapy, cognitive-behavioral interventions, eye movement desensitization and reprocessing (EMDR), sensorimotor psychotherapy, internal family systems (IFS), and, finally, mindfulness, over the course of a long and complex treatment. None of these approaches worked for long. Holly's psychopharmacologist was similarly young and dedicated and tried giving Holly virtually every antidepressant he knew. After years of concerted efforts, her treaters felt they had become a cross between cheerleaders and samurai warriors in their efforts to help Holly have a better life. However, her "treatment-resistant" depression really was treatment resistant. "I'm like Humpty Dumpty," Holly said, "I'm just too broken for therapy."

After yet another hospitalization, when Holly talked again about how broken she was, her exhausted therapist shared a story she had read about the meditation master Ajahn Chah. During a talk, he held up a beautiful crystal goblet that he was drinking from.

> You see this goblet? For me, this glass is already broken. I enjoy it; I drink out of it. It holds my water admirably, sometimes even reflecting the sun in beautiful patterns. If I should tap it, it has a lovely ring to it. But when I put this glass on a shelf and the wind knocks it over or my elbow brushes it off the table and it falls to the ground and shatters, I say, 'Of course.'

As psychiatrist Mark Epstein explains, he wasn't just speaking about the glass, "the body, or the inevitability of death. He was also speaking to each of us about the self. This self that you take to be so real, he was saying, is already broken" (Epstein, 1995, p. 81).

While this story is generally seen as a metaphor for the impermanence of all things and the constructed nature of the self, Holly heard it differently. She experienced an empathic resonance and her eyes filled with tears. "Finally, after all these years, you got it. This is what I have been trying to tell you over and over. You didn't believe me. I'm broken." Both Holly and her therapist sat in stillness for a while. Her therapist realized that her most important task at the moment was to stay with Holly's experience. "You're right," her therapist responded after a long silence. "Maybe I didn't get how broken you are. I understand that now. I can't fix you. And I do care deeply." This marked a turning point in the treatment. Holly looked stunned. "You know what? When you said that, I realized that no one, *ever*, not my mother or father or brother, ever admitted that they weren't right. No one even admitted they were fallible. That means a lot to me."

Once Holly felt truly seen, heard, and acknowledged, she stopped fighting so much and things began to shift. As Carl Rogers (1961) said, "The curious paradox of life is that when I accept myself just as I am, then I can change" (p. 17). During the next few years, Holly changed jobs, finding work that was more in tune with her values, and entered a relationship with a partner who appreciated Holly's intelligence and biting humor, matching it with her own. While she still struggled with depression, she no longer felt profoundly alone during her depressive episodes. Her caregivers had stayed with her over the long haul and were delighted as she began to find contentment and balance in midlife. All agreed that she was ready to "graduate" from psychotherapy, at least for the time being. When she turned 65, she felt that she had finally created a meaningful life for herself. "At least we don't have to continue this in the nursing home," she joked.

Ironically, the turning point in treatment had occurred when Holly heard a Buddhist teaching story in a decidedly non-Buddhist way. And she never did take to meditation.

PUTTING IT ALL TOGETHER

Every patient is different, so the ways we conduct a given hour of mindfulness-based treatment will vary greatly. Some patients will benefit from actually engaging in mindfulness practices for much of the session, others from using the last 15 or 20 minutes for practice, and yet others will do best practicing mindfulness for a few minutes at the beginning just to leave aside "road noise" and come more fully into the room. Our task is to learn how to respond as skillfully as possible to patients' changing needs.

What might an entire course of treatment look like? Which practices might we use? How do we decide? Can this be done within the constraints of managed care? What if we make a mistake? What if it doesn't work?

Short-Term Treatment of Depression

We offer the following case, just six sessions long, as an example of how treatment might unfold. Since each patient's motivation, interest, personality, and diagnosis will differ, this is simply one way treatment might be structured.

CLINICAL ILLUSTRATION: MINDFULNESS UNDER MANAGED CARE

Intake

Tim was a thin, frail young man in his late 20s, living at home and feeling stuck in his life. Witty and intense, with a gift for language, he had attended college but was currently unemployed, trying to find work as an actor while waiting on tables to pay rent to his mother. Tim's chief complaint was that he felt depressed and numb most of the time. He was not sleeping well and used over-the-counter sleeping medication to calm himself. He had been in therapy for depression in high school, which had helped, and he wanted to try again.

Tim's childhood and adolescence were dominated by a difficult relationship with his father, whom he both loved and loathed. His father, who suffered from untreated bipolar illness, had been physically abusive and was alternately charming and charismatic, angry and controlling. He had died suddenly of a massive heart attack 5 years before, but Tim had never mourned his death. "Good riddance," he felt. His parents divorced when he was in college, his mother finally finding the courage to leave after years of physical and emotional abuse.

Tim's interpersonal relationships were sparse and he had struggled with his sexual orientation. He had been in an intimate relationship for over a year, but it seemed hollow and he felt unseen. He regularly swallowed his anger and had trouble expressing his needs. He enjoyed playing other characters when he was on stage, but had difficulty being authentic in his own life. It was hard for him to be in his own skin and inhabit his own body. Tim had taken meditation classes as a way to help him cope with his depression and find some stability. Recently he had developed a knot in his stomach and pressure in his chest that worried him. He thought it might be psychosomatic and sought out a clinician who would incorporate mindfulness into his treatment.

Session 1

The first session consisted primarily of history taking and risk assessment. But toward the end of the hour, after Tim had shared some details of his father's rage, his therapist checked to see whether he was open to trying a short meditation to help him feel more grounded and come back to the present moment. "Yes, please," he said, "I always get upset talking about my childhood." The therapist started with *Simply Listening* (see Chapter 4, page 68). As Tim already had a meditation practice, he was open to turning his attention to *Finding the Breath* (see Chapter 4, page 73) after listening to sounds. As he did this, he remarked on how constricted his chest felt. He practiced staying with the sensations, not judging and not pushing them away. The area around his lungs felt like a heavy weight. Tim described it as darkness combined with a feeling of nausea.

When those sensations became too intense and painful, Tim's therapist guided him back to listening to sounds, returning to the breath when it felt safe. "It feels like there is no light, no air inside for me." He became aware of a deep sadness, first feeling it in his eyes and then his chest. This was scary for him, but with support he could bear it. As he stayed with the sensations, allowing them to come and go, his therapist wove in the suggestion, "Let me be with this . . . it's OK to feel it . . . it will pass." As Tim sat with the constriction and sadness, he commented, "It's like a prison in here—cold, gray, and the food is bad. I have been here so long. I want to stop punishing myself."

Tim's homework for the week was to bring awareness to his breath and body sensations during the day and to return to listening to sounds if he needed this as an anchor.

Session 2

Tim was able to practice a few times during the course of the week, but he didn't want to go into a frightening place alone. "My mind is a dangerous place," he quipped. The feeling of constriction and being imprisoned stayed with him. So he kept things simple, just feeling the inhalation and exhalation of the breath.

His therapist started this session with the practice of *Touch Points* (see Chapter 4, page 70), as a way to learn to ground and stabilize when difficult emotions arose. Tim reported that his body alternated between feeling sore and numb. He was interested in exploring this further, so his therapist suggested they try a guided *Compassionate Body Scan* meditation (see Chapter 6, page 105). As Tim scanned his body, beginning with his face, he noticed that he wanted to hide. "I expect to get slugged," he said. He was able to stay with this, feeling the sensations in his body, noticing tightness and clenching in his jaw and throat. He got in touch with the knot in his stomach, which was one of the feelings that had brought him back into therapy. His therapist asked him to bring awareness to the emotions behind the sensations. "I'm so used to being attacked," Tim noticed, "this knot feels like an old wound that never healed." By staying with the sensations he was able to bring kind attention to the memories of pain and abuse. He was surprised by how much tension was stored in his body. "I spent so much of my childhood afraid of getting walloped, I guess I'm still carrying that." Whenever waves of emotion or sadness arose, Tim practiced noticing them, not judging, and then letting them go. His father's verbal taunts returned as well. "He would call me a puny sissy and tell me he was beating me to toughen me up." It was painful to go back, but a relief not to be with the memories alone. "I've kept this inside, hermetically sealed for a long, long time. It's good to let some light and air into this prison."

Session 3

It had been a difficult week. Tim had had trouble sleeping and his lower back pain, an old symptom, had returned. "I feel like a sick kid." Being sick was how he got his mother's attention when he was a child. But along with it came his father's disdain. Even though he knew it would be difficult, he was ready to turn toward the sharp points. To help Tim connect with the pain but not get overwhelmed by it, his therapist taught him the practice of *Labeling Emotions* (see Chapter 5, page 94). While at first he thought his back pain was unremitting, as he paid attention to the sensations he noticed how varied they were—at first sharp, then hot, then dull and achy. At some moments there was no pain at all. Underneath the pain he began to be aware of rage, and what he described as a pure, raw terror. With this came waves of nausea. "It's like the scream in Munch's painting is in my body."

Tim stayed with these feelings, labeling them as warmly and kindly as possible, "Terror, terror, terror," and then "Nausea, nausea, nausea." Psychiatrist Dan Siegel (2010b) says that we "name it to tame it" (p. 16), and Tim found this to be true. "When I name it I find that I can be with it; it isn't so terrible." As a child, there was no way to protect himself from, or even put a name to, his father's explosive rage. So he was constantly on guard, trained to detect the slightest variation in his father's moods, never able to relax at home.

At the end of the session he felt exhausted and spent, but also had an appreciation for his courage in facing his demons. "I feel like there is some wisdom here," he said, pointing to his body. "Before I just blamed myself as weak and thought it was self-pity. I know where that story comes from," he smiled. His homework was to continue to work with the practice of *Labeling Emotions*.

Session 4

Tim practiced this meditation between sessions. He also started to write poetry about his father. Poetry was something that was not allowed in the family—it too was for "sissies." "Besides, I was so busy hating him and dreading him that I couldn't see anything else. He was such a complex and tortured man."

Tim reported that he was feeling less numb and his chest was less constricted, but the sadness was still present, as was the knot in his stomach. As he stayed with the sadness, paying attention to the sensations, he began for the first time to cry, softly at first, and then with huge, gasping sobs. "He was so terrifying at times, and yet he was my father. I've never cried like this, ever. It wasn't OK to be sad in my family. It meant you were weak and that wasn't tolerated." As he let himself feel the pain and sadness, the knot in his stomach began to soften. He stayed with it, feeling a softening in his entire body. "When I was growing up my best friend was my dog. She was a mutt that we rescued; she had been the runt of the litter. She gave me so much comfort. There was so much missing in my family."

Tim's homework was to stay with the sadness and fear and when he felt it, to note "sadness arising" or "fear arising," and to create space for these difficult emotions.

Session 5

Tim reported sleeping better and feeling lighter, more alive. "I feel like I began to pay attention and listen to all that was contained in the knot. I used to just run from it, turning to painkillers and drugs." In this session, to support and deepen this new connection with his body and sense of aliveness, his therapist suggested he try some *Walking Meditation* (see Chapter 5, page 84). "I hated my body because I was never a strong, natural athlete like my dad. I was never good enough, big enough." Walking meditation helped Tim to feel a sense of peace and confidence in his body. Simply experiencing each step, while letting thoughts come and go, made him appreciate that his body naturally knew how to walk. It didn't need to be big and tough to be valuable.

Seeing how hard it was for Tim to feel self-acceptance, his therapist next introduced *Offering Loving-Kindness to Oneself* practice (see Chapter 6, page 103), starting with sending kindness to a drama teacher in middle school who had been supportive of Tim's acting talent. "He made me feel that I was worthwhile, that I had value." When he tried to send loving-kindness to himself for the pain he was in, it seemed "alien." Being kind to oneself, he explained, was a mark of self-indulgence. After brainstorming to find some phrases that would be useful, Tim decided he liked the following: *May I be safe and protected from inner and outer harm. May I be free from loathing, disgust, and self-hatred. May I learn to be kind to myself. May I learn to care for and appreciate my body.* Tim used these phrases during the week, and added the informal practice of putting a warm hand on the knot in his stomach whenever he felt discomfort. He found this simple touch comforting: "I realize how much I stuffed it all. And I still stuff it when I'm upset. Sometimes I eat a whole pint of ice cream to soothe myself. And then I hate myself for my indulgence and lack of discipline and want to punish myself. It's good to see that cycle." His therapist added a practice to help with blame, suggesting that Tim say, "Not me, not mine, not who I am." Tim reported that this helped him realize that he was more than his symptoms.

Session 6

Tim's insurance allowed only six sessions. In this last session, he reported that for the first time in many years he felt glad to be alive. He was thinking of moving to another part of the country and trying to find an acting job. He didn't want to live with his mother anymore and figured he could wait tables in a new city. "I feel like I was living in an arid desert, and now there is finally rain, luscious drops, and air! The knot was a place of deep grief, where I didn't want to go. I feel sadness and joy, peace and excitement." As he began to wrap up and look at the work of the past sessions, Tim commented, "This is deep. I can come back to this, absorb it, and finally move on." He added with a smile, "I want to go dancing, and I was always terrified of dancing."

Tim's case is unusual in that most patients don't make this much progress in just six sessions; therapy rarely unfolds so quickly and effectively. The following case, which details the sequencing of a treatment for anxiety, is more typical in that it involves a fair amount of trial and error before any progress begins to take place.

Medium-Term Treatment of Intense Anxiety

Mindfulness can be a very useful tool in the treatment of anxiety (Roemer & Orsillo, 2009, 2013). As we open ourselves directly to the sensations, thoughts, and judgments surrounding our fears, they often become less frightening. When we begin to know and befriend our internal landscape, we can find new ways to simply be with our experience.

CLINICAL ILLUSTRATION: WAITING FOR THE NEXT DISASTER

Fatima, a school teacher in her late 30s, entered treatment because of her chronic, sometimes crippling anxiety. During the intake, Fatima said that the world never felt safe. Her father had declared bankruptcy when she was in grade school and the family had been thrown into turmoil. To make matters worse, her mother, an anxious driver, survived a serious car accident but was never quite the same. To get by during this hard time, the family was forced to live with Fatima's grandparents. She was always waiting for the next disaster to happen.

In the early stages of the treatment, Fatima was able to engage with her therapist, but had no interest in mindfulness. The only way she had of soothing herself was by running. In a few months, after developing a stronger, more trusting treatment alliance, her therapist tried again, this time mentioning the research on mindfulness and anxiety. Fatima was now more open to her therapist's suggestions. Her therapist thought *Walking Meditation* (Chapter 5, page 84) would be a good way to start, but Fatima rejected it as "boring." Building on Fatima's strengths, her therapist suggested instead that she experiment with running meditation, feeling the soles of her feet as they hit the pavement. This was promising—it helped her feel strong while the aerobic exercise lifted her mood. From there, Fatima was open to the idea of yoga to alleviate the tightness that developed after running. She explored different types, settling on a rigorous *vinyasa* flow that taught her to become aware of the sensations in her body. She learned to stay with discomfort without panicking, realizing that she could breathe through the often uncomfortable and challenging poses. "My yoga teacher says, 'No blame, no praise, just let it go.' I like that. I'm used to holding on and agonizing about things."

The focus she learned in yoga aided her concentration, and the therapist suggested the practice of *Touch Points* (see Chapter 4, page 70) and then *Compassionate Body Scan* (see Chapter 6, page 105), to build on this new ability to find safety in her body. After becoming comfortable with these practices, her therapist began to experiment with different open monitoring techniques as a way for Fatima to get curious about her anxiety (see Chapter 5). At first this was a struggle and Fatima resisted. "When I label, noting 'fear, fear,' I start worrying that I am just like my mother and I don't want to be like her," Fatima protested. "She is so pathetic!" "This is grist for the mill," her therapist responded, "I think we are seeing the underlying pattern. Let's stay curious about what is coming up for you."

In this middle stage of treatment, her therapist helped Fatima develop what meditation teachers call "nonidentification." While Fatima thought of herself as a "a ball of nerves," she realized that if she bumped her knee she didn't think of herself as a sore knee. Seeing that she was able to watch and witness thoughts helped her disentangle from her view of herself as an anxious person. Sharon Salzberg (2011) has students imagine each "thought as a visitor knocking at the door of their house. The thoughts don't live there; you greet them, acknowledging them, and watch them go" (p. 111). Realizing that this was possible allowed Fatima to bring attention to her thoughts and symptoms without making them worse. It was a relief to realize that she was more than her anxious thoughts.

Her therapist next suggested that Fatima send compassion to herself for having anxious thoughts. She particularly delighted in the *Compassionate Being* practice (see Chapter 6, page 112). Growing up in a family that thought religion was divisive, she couldn't come up with a religious or spiritual figure that spoke to her. However, her grandfather had been kind and loving. When the family lost their house after her father's bankruptcy, they lived with him until her father was back on his feet. As she practiced this meditation, she was able to access his wise and loving presence. "I always felt safe when he was around. He was such a kind and wise man. He always said that we would find a way and he was right."

Toward the end of the treatment, Fatima learned how to combine the *Compassionate Being* practice with equanimity phrases: *May I live with balance. May I have peace. May I have perspective.* Fatima had described her anxiety by saying that she felt like she was trapped in a cramped basement. She couldn't make her anxiety go away, but she could change her relationship to it. "It's like getting out of the closet and suddenly seeing that the night sky is full of stars. Yes, there are storms, there is thunder and lightning, bad things happen, but it passes. And the world is vast. When I can remember that, my anxieties don't seem nearly as big. They don't go away, but I have more perspective."

When Fatima found herself navigating rush hour traffic with less panic, she was ready to take a break from treatment. "I had structured my whole life so I didn't have to drive in the morning or at night. My world had become so small and so rigid. I still get those 'intense sensations' as we call them, but I have learned to breathe through them and they pass." Fatima's therapist supported her gains and let her know that "the door is open" if she needed to return to do another piece of work in the future.

Long-Term Treatment of Complex Trauma

The following case details recovery from severe, complex trauma. Mindfulness can be especially effective when working with trauma (Briere, 2012, 2013). Learning to stay in the present moment helps patients manage intrusive thoughts and feelings without getting stuck in the past. Loving-kindness and compassion practices can help soothe the body and connect the individual to the suffering of others.

CLINICAL ILLUSTRATION: THE PAST IS NEVER DEAD—IT'S NOT EVEN PAST

Zoe entered therapy with a history of severe and multiple traumas—a gang rape in childhood, witnessing domestic violence between her parents, and her own physical abuse by her violent, alcoholic father. Her mother, who was alternately psychotic and drug addicted, was institutionalized when Zoe was in elementary school. Her father couldn't cope with the burden of raising five children alone. Zoe and her siblings were often unwashed and neglected, fighting among themselves for limited resources, eating cold cereal for dinner when their father was in the local bar.

Since Zoe had been betrayed and abandoned from an early age, she didn't initially trust her male therapist. She had survived by her wits and her ability to fly below the radar to avoid further violence and abuse. Now in her early 30s, she had struggled with substance abuse, the sadness of an abortion, and a string of failed and abusive relationships. The world felt completely unsafe. Her therapist therefore constructed a treatment plan that integrated mindfulness meditation with an understanding of the stages of trauma and recovery, in this case using a model outlined by Judith Lewis Herman (1992).

Haunted by nightmares and flashbacks in the early stages of therapy, Zoe found it difficult to attend to the present moment or to be comfortable in her body. She complained that she wanted to "jump out of her skin" and couldn't sit still. The first therapeutic task, which took many months, was the slow process of building a trusting relationship. Once a good alliance was established, her therapist suggested *Walking Meditation* (see Chapter 5, page 84), feeling that a practice using a coarse object of attention, distant from her head and torso, would be the safest and easiest way to start (see Chapter 1). This is what Zoe turned to when she couldn't sit still. Learning to feel safe without drugs, alcohol, or sex took many more months, and was supplemented by 12-step meetings. Initially, without the self-medication of the drugs and alcohol, her flashbacks, nightmares, and night terrors intensified. When she couldn't sleep, she would practice *Walking Meditation* in the darkness of her apartment, focusing on the soles of her feet.

To help Zoe stayed grounded, her therapist next experimented with the *Touch Points* (see Chapter 4, page 70), starting from the feet up instead of the head down, to make it feel safer. This helped Zoe with her frequent, often overwhelming, panic. She practiced sequentially bringing attention to her feet, knees, sitting bones, hands, hips, and eyes.

During this stage of establishing safety, Zoe also tried the practice of *Simply Listening* (see Chapter 4, page 68), using the noise of the city as an object of awareness. Cars, voices, even fire engines and ambulances made her feel less alone and less frightened that her violent father would return to harm her. The phrase *If it isn't happening now, it isn't happening* helped her stay in the present moment and manage her panic and dissociation. After more than 2 years of therapy, mindfulness practices, and 12-step meetings, Zoe was in a safe living situation, was sober, and had returned to school to get a college degree.

After establishing safety, the next stage of recovery in Herman's (1992) model is "Remembrance and Mourning," which characterized the middle phase of the treatment. Zoe continued to remember and talk about the abuse she had suffered. However, as she began to mourn and remember, her symptoms intensified again. It became hard for her to get out of bed. Although her therapist tried introducing compassion practice, Zoe was not ready for this, partly believing her mother's words that she was "the devil's spawn." This period of therapy was arduous, marked by frequent setbacks, relapses, and health problems. Zoe did her best to manage her symptoms, but she sometimes pushed the boundaries of the treatment: canceling at the last minute, storming out of sessions, and skipping an appointment if she didn't feel "in the mood." When her therapist set limits, she flew into a rage, accused him of being just "like my father," and fired him—although she returned with apologies the following week. Her therapist, realizing that he was in over his head, sought additional consultation for himself, while connecting Zoe with a psychoeducational group for trauma survivors. Both Zoe and her therapist took comfort in the fact that they could both start again and again and again. Her therapist found personal and professional sustenance himself by joining a supervision group for clinicians working with trauma.

In this challenging stage of treatment, lasting nearly 3 years, the practice of *Labeling Emotions* (see Chapter 5, page 94) became Zoe's refuge when things got rough. She found that "putting a frame" around her negative, ruminative thoughts helped her get through dark times. She would practice letting the thoughts arise, noting them, and then returning attention to the soles of her feet if she felt overwhelmed. When she began to think, "I'm a worthless failure," she would label the thought as "failure" and feel the sensations that accompanied it. She noticed tightness in her jaw and a pit in her stomach. With effort and concentration, Zoe was able to identify a repeating pattern—when sensations and thoughts related to failure arose, she thought, "I need to get out of here," "I need a drink," or "I need sex." Seeing this sequence of sensations, thoughts, and impulses helped her begin to break the destructive pattern.

At times Zoe got caught in what she called a "hurricane of hatred."

Re-introducing compassion practices (see Chapter 6), her therapist explained that many survivors of abuse have trouble feeling compassion for themselves. Zoe realized that she felt more comfortable sending loving-kindness to others. Beginning here, Zoe gradually learned to include herself in the circle of care. She experimented with creating her own version of a self-compassion break (chapter 6, page 107), saying to herself: "OK, you're in pain right now. Stay present. Everyone screws up. You haven't killed or maimed anyone. Stay with it, get curious about it." She then added: *May I be free from hatred. May I be free from despair. May I be free from the past. May I be free from my childhood.*

Zoe eventually finished school and found a job as a counselor in a woman's shelter. Continuing in therapy and now taking meditation classes at her local adult education center, she was ready to work on the final stage of recovery, which Herman (1992) calls "Reconnection." While there was no way to comprehend her senseless childhood gang rape, she could begin to understand the profound limitations of her mother (now dead) and gain insights into her father's violent rage. He was currently living in a nursing home, partially paralyzed by a stroke. No longer menacing, he was a frail, sick, old man. Her older siblings, who also struggled tremendously, told her how he had been victimized by his own father and older brothers. She would never condone his behavior, but she could comprehend how family life had spiraled down into chaos and violence.

As Zoe sat with her father in his dying days, she was able to revisit loving-kindness practices for herself and her troubled family: *May we all be safe. May we all be healthy. May we treat one another with kindness. May we remember that we can always begin again.*

Zoe didn't expect to stay with her father as he died. She planned to pay her respects and go home. But he was sicker than she thought and she realized that she wanted closure. As she listened to his labored breathing, she practiced the *Mountain Meditation* (see Chapter 7, page 122), aware of the passing of time, the storms of rage and violence that had subsided, and his withered body gasping for its last few breaths. "I'm glad I stayed. I never thought I would say this, but it was good for me to see that the monster had become a frightened and helpless old man." A friend at the shelter where she worked had given her a poem by Tony Hoagland (2003) that she read over and over at her father's bedside: The following lines spoke to her:

> Maybe I overdid it
> when I called my father an enemy of humanity . . .
> What I meant was that my father
> was an enemy of my humanity . . .

living deep inside of me
like a bad king or an incurable disease—blighting my crops, striking
    down my herds, poisoning my wells . . .
I don't want to scream forever
I don't want to live without proportion
like some kind of infection from the past. . . ." (p. 40)*

The work with Zoe continues.

Mindful Termination

From the perspective of mindfulness-oriented therapy, the word *termination* is a bit of a misnomer, for mindfulness practice and work on oneself never ends—it is the work of a lifetime. Zen masters use the image of continuously polishing a mirror. As mindfulness grows and troubling symptoms subside, it is not that one is ever finished or "cured," but more likely that insurance coverage has ended, the crisis has passed, or enough balance has been achieved that one can take a break from therapy and return to the business of living one's life. The Sufi story of Mullah Nasruddin illustrates this point: A proud mother announced, "My son has finished his studies." Nasruddin replied, "No doubt God will send him more" (Kornfield, 2000, p. 112). Developing concentration, mindfulness, loving-kindness, compassion, and equanimity is an ongoing practice. Meditation teachers like to joke that there is no "enlightened retirement."

When we accept patients into our practice, we generally make a commitment to be a resource for as long as they need us, if possible. We have a number of patients who began treatment in high school, college, or early adulthood who return when they hit "bumps" in the road of life. In this model, we think of the relationship between the therapist and patient as a fluid one, an enduring connection over time that allows the patient to come and go as needed.

Many factors influence the rhythm of treatment, including when and how we reduce its intensity. While there are valid arguments for underscoring the end of treatment as a way to rework feelings about separation and loss, sometimes, when it seems that a patient will benefit from ongoing support and we're able to provide it, treatment doesn't so much end as taper.

---

* Copyright 2003 by Tony Hoagland. Reprinted by permission.

CLINICAL ILLUSTRATION: WINDING DOWN

It had been one painful event after another for Antonio. His lover of
many years left him for a younger man, he lost his job in advertising
after an important client was critical of his work, and his mother was
fading into a fog of dementia. "She smiles politely when I visit, but
she has no clue who I am," Antonio said with tears in his eyes. Now
that he was out of work, he wanted to take an extended vacation and
visit friends while figuring out his next step, but he didn't feel that he
could abandon his mother. "I don't know how much longer she has
and I don't want to spend the rest of my life feeling guilty. She was
there for me after I came out about my sexuality, even though she
believed it was a sin and my father disowned me. That took real guts,"
he sighed. "I know, I speak of her in the past, but she certainly isn't in
the present."

Antonio complained of feeling anxious and depressed. Lacking
the structure of work, he was partying and drinking too much. He
was open to trying mindfulness in addition to talk therapy. Since he
was relatively stable and self-aware, his therapist taught him to bring
his attention to his breath (see Chapter 4), which he liked. Feeling
easily distracted, he especially enjoyed a variation where he counted
backward from four to one, counting four on the inhalation and the
exhalation, then three on the inhalation and the exhalation, then two,
etc. "It takes a little more effort than counting to 10 and my mind
wanders less."

In therapy, as he talked about the end of his relationship, previously disavowed emotions flooded back into awareness: "When I think
about Matthew, I want him to hurt too. I've never felt this angry. I
feel like I'm a bad, horrible creature." His therapist encouraged him to
allow these negative emotions to arise. "Unpleasant feelings are every
bit as important as positive ones. They help us to understand and be
honest about our experience," he explained. Rather than bury them,
his therapist taught him to recognize when he was agitated or upset,
using the practice of *Labeling Emotions* (see Chapter 5, page 94) to
maintain perspective. Antonio began by noticing "revenge, revenge"
and "rage, rage." This was a challenge. "In my family, we didn't do
negative emotions. My father would yell at me if I looked angry." As
they worked together, Antonio began to accept anger as part of life.
"It's like an early warning system; it's a sign that I need to pay attention,
that something isn't working."

As his symptoms began to abate, Anthony found it comforting
to practice a variation on *tonglen* (see Chapter 6, page 116) where he
breathed in compassion for his pain and distress, and breathed out

compassion for others who have been betrayed, hurt, or whose loved ones are ill or dying (see the Appendix for this variation).

After over a year of weekly treatment, Antonio was less distressed and he and his therapist agreed to taper the treatment, initially meeting every other week and then meeting monthly. He had entered a new relationship, "rather vanilla ice cream but we are good for each other," and started a new job: "It pays the rent and there is room to grow." His cynical edge softened when he spoke of his mother, "Sometimes when I visit I just sit with her and practice *Breathing Together* (see Chapter 3, page 60). Yesterday, she reached out and touched my cheek. She hasn't done anything like that in a long time. She doesn't talk, but we sit together in silence. And those moments feel like a blessing."

Despite doing considerably better, and feeling that his life was basically on track, Antonio didn't want to end therapy. "Knowing we'll meet helps me continue my mindfulness practice, and reminds me that my anger is OK. And I value our connection." His therapist let Antonio set the pace of treatment. Most recently they've been meeting three to four times a year, and Antonio continues to feel that his life is moving in a positive direction.

Of course, other treatments have clearer endpoints, either for practical reasons or because the therapist and patient recognize that a more formal ending would provide an opportunity to explore important feelings associated with separation and loss. An important goal of such terminations is to help the patient carry forward supportive memories of the therapist and the therapy process.

When it's finally time to say good-bye, we've found the following exercise can facilitate this consolidation. It was inspired by a practice taught by Emily Schatzow and Judith Lewis Herman as a way to honor an individual's "graduation" from a trauma and recovery group. We have adapted it here for individual treatment.

MINDFUL TERMINATION: AN ACCOUNT OF THE JOURNEY

Before the final session, the therapist reviews his or her notes, looking at the course of treatment—where the patient started, what issues were explored, what challenges were overcome, and what insights occurred. The therapist then writes a paragraph or two about the journey. Finally, he or she reads these words aloud and gives them to the patient in a note.

We have found that these few paragraphs become a meaningful document, and that most patients save the note. Some access it during difficult times. Especially for patients who had inadequate primary relationships, to know that someone has witnessed, seen, and cared about their suffering is a source of sustenance.

CLINICAL ILLUSTRATION:
MINDFULNESS AND COMPASSION ARE ALWAYS AVAILABLE

Natasha had grown up with neglect as well as physical and emotional abuse. While her insurance covered only a brief treatment, it was a radical and reparative experience to receive kindness, warmth, and compassion from her therapist. It was especially helpful for her to have a list of the mindfulness practices that were introduced in treatment. The ending note became a "transitional object"; it reminded her that she wasn't alone, that she could start again and return to her practice if she had taken a "break." For Natasha, the note was a resource, and a reminder that she could live a life of mindfulness, compassion, and equanimity—it was as close as her next breath.

CHAPTER TEN

Beyond Symptom Relief

Deepening Mindfulness

But those who follow the dharma, when it has been well taught, will reach the other shore, hard to reach, beyond the realm of death.

—THE BUDDHA (in Easwaran, 2007, p. 127)

What is the goal of psychotherapy? What do patients seek when they come in for treatment? What exactly do we as psychotherapists offer them? And does the goal line shift when we introduce mindfulness meditation? In the short term, the goals of meditation and psychotherapy appear quite similar. Both offer relief from suffering. Both promise insights that can lead to improved mood and greater self-acceptance. Both help people understand and change habitual, self-defeating patterns in the ways they think, behave, and relate to others. But when we look further down the road, we can see that while these two disciplines both offer the potential for emotional and psychological healing, they can ultimately lead to two very different destinations.

175

In this final chapter, we examine some of the issues that emerge when our patients are ready to move beyond the treatment of symptoms toward a deeper exploration of what it means to lead happier, more meaningful lives. In the process, we revisit some of the ideas and themes mentioned earlier in the book, such as developing our own (and our patients') meditation practice, participating in retreats, and working with philosophical teachings that are associated with mindfulness and meditation. We also examine some of these teachings from the perspective of their original purpose.

Psychotherapy is primarily about helping people reduce mental suffering so that they can lead more productive, satisfying lives. For those of us who deal with insurance companies and managed care, this means restoring our patients to higher levels of social and occupational functioning as quickly and efficiently as possible. From this point of view, the consulting room can feel like an army field hospital, where we patch people up as best we can and send them back into the fray. Not that there's anything wrong with that. In fact, it's what most patients need and want, and what many of today's clinicians hope to deliver. Even Sigmund Freud (Freud & Breuer, 1893-1895/2000), who could hardly be accused of employing a short-term or superficial approach, famously (and modestly) said that his methods were designed to transform "hysterical misery into common unhappiness" so that his patients could be "better armed against that unhappiness" (p. 305)— not exactly a lofty goal.

Meditation aims considerably higher, and most people know it. Even those who say that the only reason they'll try meditation is to reduce their stress, relieve their lower back pain, or fall asleep at night, probably have at least some inkling of what the Buddha discovered some 2,600 years ago. It's variously called nirvana, enlightenment, the deathless, or the unconditioned. And while it's impossible to describe in words, it involves a radical transformation of consciousness that not only changes our understanding of who we are and how we're connected with the rest of the cosmos but also—if the ancient texts are to be believed—brings mental suffering to a complete and permanent end (see Fulton & Siegel, 2013, for a detailed comparison of Buddhist and Western psychological traditions).

If we believe such a transformation is possible, then that will almost certainly have an effect on how we understand our role as mindfulness-informed psychotherapists.

ARE WE THERAPISTS OR MEDITATION TEACHERS?

This is a question many therapists begin to ask themselves once they start incorporating meditation and other mindfulness practices into their work. The line between mental health professional and meditation teacher can easily become blurred, and this can be a problem. Very few therapists have the depth of meditative experience and understanding required of a skilled meditation teacher. What's more, in the secular world of psychotherapy, especially when third-party payers are involved, we therapists may feel obligated to stay in our therapist chairs and to use meditative techniques only for the purpose of relieving psychiatric symptoms.

But what if our patients want to go deeper? What if they come in with existential questions about impermanence and the nature of the self? These concerns can lead to some interesting clinical and ethical dilemmas. And while there are no simple answers, there are two things we can do that will almost always serve us and our patients well: deepen our own meditation practice and encourage our patients to deepen theirs.

DEEPENING OUR OWN MEDITATION PRACTICE

In Chapter 2, we stressed the importance of developing our own mindfulness meditation practice before beginning to offer mindfulness tools and techniques to patients. The more we deepen our meditation practice, the more effective we will be when we share those tools and techniques. And our effectiveness will go beyond the mere ability to teach mindfulness skills. For as we deepen our own practice, we will also begin to embody the qualities of wisdom and compassion that are so essential in a skilled psychotherapist (Germer & Siegel, 2012).

So how do we deepen our understanding of mindfulness in order to grow in both wisdom and compassion? There are basically three ways: practicing, studying, and connecting with others.

Maintaining a Daily Practice

Setting the intention to sit every day, or at least most days, is crucial. One of our colleagues calls it "mental floss," a daily cleaning that helps us let go of mental preoccupations, anchor the mind in the present moment, and make the shift from "doing mode" to "being mode" (Segal et al., 2002; Segal, Williams, & Teasdale, 2012). We can further enliven our practice by challenging ourselves to sit for longer periods and to move beyond concentration to incorporate open monitoring, loving-kindness, compassion, equanimity, and the related practices described in this book. Consulting with a qualified meditation teacher can also be a great help, as can reading books about meditation and listening to guided meditations and dharma talks (see the Resources).

Taking the Plunge: Exploring Retreat Practice

As we first mentioned in Chapter 1, going on a meditation retreat is a powerful way to deepen our experience of mindfulness as well as our understanding of how the mind creates suffering for itself. Of course, packing up and heading off for a multiday retreat can be daunting for logistical as well as emotional reasons. But most who have done it agree that sitting a retreat can be a profound experience, and many mindfulness-informed psychotherapists consider retreat practice an essential part of their training and continuing education.

If you've never been on a retreat, you may wonder exactly what goes on there. Different meditative traditions have created various forms and structures for the retreat experience, but they tend to have much in common. Retreats are generally held in silence, except for brief periods when questions are allowed either in a group setting or in individual meetings with the teacher. Many centers ask participants to follow training precepts such as refraining from causing harm to any living being, refraining from misuse of speech (on retreat, this usually means not speaking at all), refraining from taking anything that is not freely given, refraining from sexual misconduct, and refraining from the use of intoxicants. They sometimes also include a daily period of mindful work. And they usually include an extensive schedule of formal meditation practice from early in the morning until late in the evening.

Typical Retreat Schedule

Here's a typical daily schedule for a retreat at the Insight Meditation Society, a well-known vipassana (insight) meditation retreat center in Barre, Massachusetts:

5:30 A.M.   Wake up
6:00 A.M.   Sitting meditation

6:30 A.M.	Breakfast
7:15 A.M.	Work-as-practice period
8:15 A.M.	Sitting meditation with instructions
9:15 A.M.	Walking meditation
10:00 A.M.	Sitting meditation
10:45 A.M.	Walking meditation or interviews with teachers
11:30 A.M.	Sitting meditation
12:00 noon	Lunch
1:45 P.M.	Walking meditation
2:15 P.M.	Sitting meditation
3:00 P.M.	Walking meditation
3:45 P.M.	Sitting meditation
4:30 P.M.	Walking meditation
5:00 P.M.	Light dinner
6:15 P.M.	Sitting meditation
7:00 P.M.	Walking meditation
7:30 P.M.	Dharma talk
8:30 P.M.	Walking meditation
9:00 P.M.	Sitting meditation
9:30 P.M.	Late tea, further practice or sleep

If a weeklong residential retreat sounds too ambitious, you may want to get your feet wet by trying a shorter, nonresidential retreat first. Many urban retreat centers offer 1-day or 2-day retreats, which are usually held on weekends. These retreats follow a similar daily schedule, but they start later in the morning, and in the evening the participants go home or to a local hotel to sleep (more on these later).

Studying Buddhist Psychology or Other Wisdom Traditions

While mindfulness meditation has been developed in many different cultural and religious contexts, many of the practices that are now being incorporated by psychotherapists come from Buddhist traditions. Here mindfulness is one part of an "eightfold path." Only three of the path's eight components—Wise Effort, Wise Mindfulness, and Wise Concentration—are specifically about meditation. Three others—Wise Speech, Wise Action, and Wise Livelihood—are concerned with ethics and our conduct in the world, and the other two—Wise View and Wise Thought—are related to the development of wisdom (Johnson, 2004).

By focusing only on meditation, mindfulness-oriented psychotherapists are sometimes accused by traditional Buddhist practitioners of missing the bigger picture and neglecting other, equally important aspects of the path to awakening. There's undoubtedly some truth to this accusation. But as discussed in Chapter 1, in clinical settings where we're working with patients who come from various religious backgrounds and who hold a wide variety of beliefs, talking about Buddhism or other religious traditions can alienate those who have different beliefs. What we can do, however, is point to the insights that naturally arise through mindfulness meditation and explore how these insights can help our patients live more wisely and reduce the amount of suffering they create for themselves and the other people in their lives.

For example, consider the teachings on the three characteristics of existence—impermanence (*anicca*), unsatisfactoriness (*dukkha*), and noself (*anatta*)—found in Buddhist traditions (see Chapter 1). Like many Buddhist teachings, these teachings aren't actually beliefs or doctrines, but observations about the mind and the world that are compatible with most of the world's great religious, spiritual, philosophic, and scientific traditions. What's more, they aren't to be taken on faith alone, but are meant to be investigated. The Buddha often exhorted his followers not to believe anything just because he (or anyone else) was proclaiming it, but to look within, pay attention, and see for themselves.

So when we practice mindfulness and look deeply, can we see the three characteristics of existence?

Well, we can probably see that everything we encounter in this world is impermanent, which not only means that things don't last but that they're constantly changing from moment to moment. We might even notice that "things" don't exist—they're constructs our mind uses to organize the flux of ever-changing experience. Modern science, from electron microscopy to particle physics, concurs.

We can also see that the mind reacts with dissatisfaction quite often. That's relatively easy to notice when what we're looking at is unpleasant. But even if it's pleasurable, we can see that it's subject to change and will eventually fade, leaving us feeling empty and wanting more. As the great philosopher-sage Roseanne Roseannadanna put it, "If it's not one thing, it's another."

Finally, and this is perhaps the hardest to observe at first, we can begin to see that nothing has "self"—an inherent or lasting core. Everything, including our own sense of self, is constantly arising and passing away from moment to moment and changing based on fluctuating internal and external conditions. During meditation, we can't find a stable little homunculus inside, nothing solid we can point to and say, "That's me."

Awakening to these three existential realities, whether we conceptualize them in Buddhist or other terms, is important for developing our insight, wisdom, and compassion (Siegel, 2012). In psychotherapy, being aware of these realities can affect how we see our patients and how we hold their suffering. Eventually it can also affect how patients see themselves and relate to their own suffering, even if we never mention Buddhist thought or the concepts of impermanence, unsatisfactoriness, and no-self. Perhaps a brief example will help illustrate how this process can work—in this case, how the therapist's awareness of no-self subtly influenced treatment.

CLINICAL ILLUSTRATION: WHOSE ANXIETY IS IT, ANYWAY?

Beatrice was a piano teacher who thoroughly enjoyed her work with her young students, but who froze whenever she was asked to play at social gatherings or with other musician friends. "I wish I could," she said, "but I'm just too anxious." In therapy, she remembered how anxious her parents became before and during her piano recitals when she was growing up, and she began to see this anxiety as a seed that was transmitted to her and grew into the anxiety that had kept her from performing as an adult. She also learned mindfulness techniques she could use at home when she was practicing the piano: bringing her attention to her breathing, her foot on the pedals, or her fingertips on the keys, as she imagined herself performing before an audience. By relating to the anxiety in a more impersonal way, her therapist helped Beatrice not identify with it so strongly. While her therapist never used the term, he helped her approach her anxiety from the perspective of no-self:

BEATRICE: I'm such an anxious person . . . I just can't stand it!

THERAPIST: Instead of seeing yourself as an anxious person, can you just see it as "anxiety arising"?

BEATRICE: No way! *I'm* the one who's feeling it.

THERAPIST: True, but is that all you're feeling? Do you always feel it? Do you feel it everywhere?

BEATRICE: No . . . mostly just when I have to play the piano in
    front of people.

THERAPIST: What are you feeling right now?

BEATRICE: Well, I'm feeling a little anxious . . . a little confused
    . . . and a little cold.

THERAPIST: Does that make you a cold person?

BEATRICE: Not necessarily . . .

Because her therapist never described what Beatrice was experiencing as "her anxiety" but instead as "the anxiety" or "anxiety arising," Beatrice gradually began to take it less personally too. She also learned to see it as a form of suffering and to send herself compassion when the anxiety was present. Eventually, she agreed to play at a birthday party for a friend. "It was OK," she reported the following week. "I could feel the anxiety, but I could also feel my fingers on the keys, listen to the sound of the music, wish myself well, and even wish the audience well. The anxiety was present, but I could see that it was just part of the whole experience."

Finding Community

In Buddhist traditions, practitioners are encouraged take refuge in the Three Gems—the Buddha, the Dharma, and the Sangha—for support along the path to awakening. Taking refuge in "the Buddha" involves taking heart: because the historical Buddha awakened, we can too. It also suggests taking refuge in the Buddha within, the one (or part of us) that knows how to awaken, that practices daily meditation and goes on retreats. "The Dharma" (or law of nature) is the body of teachings, the insights into existential reality and the workings of the mind we can reflect upon and that provide guidance along the way. Finally, "the Sangha" is the community of teachers and other like-minded individuals who can inspire us and keep us on track. Many other wisdom traditions also emphasize the importance of community support for spiritual development.

    Being part of a community is another important way to deepen both our understanding and our own meditation practice. If there's a meditation center in your area, consider getting involved. If not, see if you can form a sitting and/or study group with other mindfulness-oriented clinicians in your area. Or look for connections and other resources online. At the Institute for Meditation and Psychotherapy, we've noticed a growing need for community among therapists who are interested in integrating meditation with their clinical work and are actively involved in creating new opportunities for our members to connect with one another. (See the website *www.meditationandpsychotherapy.org* for more information.)

DEEPENING OUR PATIENTS' MEDITATION PRACTICE

Most patients will be content to deploy mindfulness skills to shift their relationship to their immediate suffering, and in the process, to enjoy some relief from symptoms of anxiety, depression, and other psychological ills. Most will not have the time, motivation, or discipline to establish and maintain a regular daily meditation practice. But some will. And some will want to go deeper—to go on retreats and explore the body of teachings from which many mindfulness practices stem. A few may even come to therapy with an active meditation practice (a "preexisting meditative condition") and a desire to work with a clinician who can help them use that practice in the service of their own emotional and spiritual growth.

So how can we best work with patients while being mindful of the line between psychotherapist and meditation teacher? The following example illustrates some possibilities.

CLINICAL ILLUSTRATION: STEPPING OFF THE TREADMILL

Charlotte was a high-powered attorney in her late 30s, working hard to make partner at a large, prestigious law firm. Happily married to a top executive at a major financial services company, she was secure financially, but was troubled by a constant undercurrent of worries about her appearance, her health, and the fact that her two young children were spending more time with their nanny than with her. Driven by her critical and overachieving family of origin, Charlotte had suffered from low-level depression and self-critical thoughts for most of her life. More recently, she had also been experiencing frequent headaches and gastrointestinal distress. Her doctor ruled out medical causes and suggested she look into ways to reduce stress, including meditation. He also gave her the name of a mindfulness-oriented psychotherapist. Since Charlotte had already dabbled with meditation when she was in college and found it useful, she was open to the idea and set up an appointment.

In therapy, Charlotte explored her personal history and learned basic mindfulness skills to help manage her day-to-day stress more effectively. But due to her busy schedule, she said she wasn't able to meditate regularly at home. And while she gained some insight and perspective on her self-critical thoughts, her depression persisted, as did her headaches and stomach problems. To deepen her practice, her therapist recommended she sign up for an 8-week MBSR program at a local hospital, and Charlotte agreed.

During the program, Charlotte resolved to do her homework and meditate just about every day for 45 minutes. Gradually, things began to improve. She learned to relate to her headaches and stomachaches with acceptance and curiosity instead of fear, and they soon became less frequent and less intense. She also deepened her ability to bring mindfulness to the negative thoughts feeding her depression and began to see them simply as thoughts—a story she was telling herself—and not necessarily the truth. When the MBSR program ended, she continued to practice at least 20 minutes a day, and also began going to classes at a local meditation center. She found herself drawn to the Buddhist teachings, and with her therapist's encouragement, decided to go on a weeklong retreat. While on retreat, she found herself questioning whether her goal of becoming a partner at her law firm was worth the cost. When she returned, she felt even more committed to the path of mindfulness, and told her therapist that her new goal was to "step off the treadmill" and find ways to cut back on her work schedule so that she could spend more time on the meditation cushion and with her kids.

Peeking Inside the Trojan Horse

What Charlotte discovered is described by our colleague Paul Fulton as the "Trojan horse" of mindfulness-based psychotherapy: Attracted by the prospect of relieving their distress, some patients begin mindfulness practice, only to realize there's a lot more to this apparently simple practice than they ever imagined.

Of course, many patients aren't inclined to look inside the Trojan horse. And that's OK. But for those who are, we mindfulness-oriented clinicians should be aware that what they find there can be both challenging and transformative. Then we can decide if we'd like to encourage further exploration by referring our patients to either a meditation center or a clinically based program where they can get more intensive mindfulness training. (Later in this chapter, we review some of the guidelines that can help us determine whether to make such a referral.)

Mindfulness Training in Clinical Settings

Over the past two decades, there's been an explosion of research showing mindfulness practice to be an effective treatment for a wide range of medical and psychiatric disorders (Germer et al., 2013). As a result, an ever-increasing number of mindfulness-based treatment programs are being developed within Western health care systems. These programs offer patients an opportunity to deepen their understanding of mindfulness practice. They typically utilize a group format, are led by clinicians or other professionals who have received special training, and are held in hospitals, mental health centers, private practices, and other clinical settings. They are usually time limited (8–10 weeks), with weekly meetings that last 2 hours or longer. Some programs also include a daylong retreat. Although they are more like meditation classes than psychotherapy groups, these programs are completely secular in nature, with few if any references to the Buddhist or other traditions from which many mindfulness practices are drawn.

What Makes Group Mindfulness Programs Effective?

In a mindfulness-based group, participants enjoy a number of advantages that are difficult, if not impossible, to offer in individual psychotherapy.

- *Focus.* The group is focused almost exclusively on the learning and practicing of mindfulness skills.
- *Depth.* Because the group meetings are longer than individual therapy sessions, participants can practice for longer periods of time and reach deeper levels of concentration and mindfulness (and have more opportunities to confront obstacles to practice).
- *Guidance.* Group leaders guide the meditations during meetings, and participants have access to recorded guided meditations they can use at home. Like training wheels, guided meditations help keep beginners on track until they are more comfortable practicing on their own.
- *Modeling.* In the way they handle participants' questions and concerns, group leaders do their best to model attention, acceptance, and compassion.

- *Homework.* Participants commit to practicing every day at home, which can be a great way to establish a daily practice and experience its benefits.
- *Peer support.* Practicing in the company of others gives participants the courage to persist through inevitable challenges, while hearing about others' struggles can normalize the difficulties they encounter.

Let's look at a few representative multicomponent, empirically supported, mindfulness-based clinical programs. These are all secular in their approach, with few mentions of spiritual or religious traditions.

Mindfulness-Based Stress Reduction

Since the late 1970s, the MBSR program has been a major force in the introduction of mindfulness practice to health care systems, educational institutions, corporations, government agencies, and thousands of individuals all over the globe. It is now available in over 30 countries on five continents. Originally developed by Jon Kabat-Zinn at the University of Massachusetts Medical School as a treatment for patients with chronic pain (Kabat-Zinn, 1982; Kabat-Zinn, Lipworth, Burney, & Sellers, 1986), MBSR has since been studied and appears to be an effective treatment for everything from anxiety (Kabat-Zinn et al., 1992) to psoriasis (Kabat-Zinn et al., 1998), and has repeatedly been shown to significantly change brain structure and function (see Lazar, 2013, for a review). The program consists of eight 2.5-hour meetings, with a full-day retreat scheduled sometime between the sixth and seventh meeting. It combines mindfulness meditation, yoga, group discussion, and other exercises to help participants transform their relationship to their distress. Participants are expected to devote at least 45 minutes to their homework each day. MBSR is a proven program that helps patients taste the benefits of having a regular daily practice and is especially effective for those with psychophysiological conditions.

Mindfulness-Based Cognitive Therapy

Mindfulness-based cognitive therapy (MBCT) was developed by researchers from England and Canada who were looking for a new way to address the problem of recurrent depression. Introduced in 2002 (Segal et al., 2002, 2012), MBCT is now offered throughout Great Britain as part of the National Health Service and is becoming increasingly available in other countries. Building on the MBSR model, MBCT adds elements of cognitive therapy to help participants apply mindfulness specifically to the symptoms of depression. But it is primarily a course in mindfulness meditation. Mark Williams, one of the developers of the program, has described it as "80% meditation, 20% cognitive therapy" (Law, 2008). The MBCT program consists of eight 2-hour group meetings, plus an initial individual assessment meeting. Participants are expected to do about 1 hour of meditation practice and other exercises each day. Follow-up group meetings are also recommended, but are not an integral part of the program. MBCT has been studied extensively and appears to be an effective treatment for recurrent depression (Ma & Teasdale, 2004; Teasdale et al., 2000). In fact, randomized controlled studies have shown MBCT to be as effective as antidepressant medication in preventing relapse, and more effective in reducing residual symptoms and improving patients' quality of life (Kuyken et al., 2008; Godfrin & van Heeringen, 2010).

Mindfulness-Based Relapse Prevention

Developed by G. Alan Marlatt and his colleagues at the University of Washington, mindfulness-based relapse prevention (MBRP) is an 8-week group program designed to help participants maintain recovery from substance abuse and other addictive behaviors. Just as MBCT was based on MBSR, MBRP is based on MBCT, in that it combines mindfulness training with techniques from cognitive therapy. In MBRP, the goal is to help participants identify triggers, habitual patterns of thought, and resulting reactions that lead to relapse. By bringing mindfulness to these destructive, seemingly automatic patterns, participants learn that they can pause, cultivate acceptance toward their troubling thoughts and feelings, and instead of continuing their addictive behaviors, make wiser choices (Bowen, Chawla, & Marlatt, 2011). One of the more popular techniques from this program is called "urge surfing," in which participants practice staying mindful of urges—waves of sensations, thoughts, and feelings that would normally compel them to use a substance—and simply ride the waves until they subside (see *Riding the Wave*, Chapter 7, page 125). Early research (Witkiewitz & Bowen, 2010) indicates that the program helps participants control and reduce craving.

Mindful Self-Compassion

Developed by Christopher Germer (2009) and Kristin Neff (2011), mindful self-compassion (MSC) is a group program that includes eight 2.5-hour weekly meetings, as well as a half-day retreat. Utilizing guided meditations, group exercises, discussion, and home practice, MSC is designed to help participants cultivate compassion for themselves. It is complementary to programs such as MBSR and MBCT that emphasize moment-to-moment awareness. Whereas mindfulness helps us open to pain and suffering with spacious awareness, self-compassion, the focus of the program, is the warmhearted attitude that arises when we meet suffering and manage to stay mindful. In a pilot randomized clinical trial of MSC, the participants who completed the program showed significant increases in self-compassion, mindfulness, compassion for others, and life satisfaction—and significant decreases in depression, anxiety, stress, and avoidance (Neff & Germer, 2012).

Many other secular mindfulness-based clinical programs have also been developed. Some, such as mindfulness-based eating awareness training (MB-EAT; Kristeller, Baer, & Quillian-Wolever, 2006) and acceptance-based behavior therapy for generalized anxiety disorder (ABBT for GAD; Orsillo & Roemer, 2011), are focused on specific conditions, whereas others, such as dialectical behavior therapy (DBT; Linehan, 1993b) and acceptance and commitment therapy (ACT; Hayes & Strosahl, 2005), are broader in focus. These programs all vary in the degree to which they include formal meditation practice. Another program of potential interest to both clinicians and patients is insight dialogue (Kramer, 2007; Surrey & Kramer, 2013), which is more explicitly rooted in Buddhist teachings and offers interpersonal mindfulness practices to help practitioners bring meditative awareness to speaking, listening, and other aspects of their relationships. (See the Resources for a more complete listing.)

Mindfulness Training in Meditation Centers

After experiencing some of the benefits of mindfulness practice, some patients will feel a natural affinity for it, and will decide to practice at a meditation center as a way of deepening their experience. With such patients, there's nothing much we need to do except, perhaps, explore with them whether or not these activities are supporting their emotional, psychological, and spiritual development.

With other patients, however, we may be tempted to encourage them to try practicing at a meditation center, to work with a qualified meditation teacher, or even to go on retreat. Maybe we sense they need more structure and discipline or would benefit from the support of a community of practitioners. Or maybe they have questions about the practice that we're just not able to answer.

But referring a patient to a meditation center should not be done lightly. Before doing so, there are a number of questions to consider, including:

• *Will the patient perceive it as proselytizing?* Since many mindfulness-informed clinicians are most familiar with Buddhist meditation centers, and since Buddhism is seen by many as a religion, certain patients will be wary. Of course, many people consider Buddhism to be a philosophical and psychological system with a body of teachings and practices that can be separated from their religious context and integrated with Western scientific or religious teachings and practices. For example, Steven Batchelor (1998, 2010) has written extensively about practicing Buddhism in a totally secular way. And most skilled Buddhist teachers are less concerned with gaining converts to a belief system than with sharing practices and ideas that will help people lead happier lives, whatever their religion happens to be. The Dalai Lama has even said that he doesn't think Westerners should become Buddhists, but should embrace the teachings on wisdom and compassion within their own religious or secular traditions. Still, many patients will simply not feel comfortable going to a Buddhist meditation center, and any suggestion that they do so could be experienced as an empathic failure, an attempt to impose alien values and beliefs, or both. For these patients, referral to a clinical program such as MBSR or to a retreat center within their own religious tradition may be most appropriate, even if the center might not teach mindfulness in the same way that we have been presenting it.

• *Is the patient up to it?* At most meditation centers, patients will not receive the kind of individual attention they get in therapy or in a mindfulness-based group in a clinical setting. And they will probably not be working with people who are trained clinicians. They may also be expected to practice for longer periods with relatively little guidance, especially during retreats. For these reasons, the intensive meditation practiced at many centers can be destabilizing for some patients, including those who have fragile or rigid personality structures, are substance dependent, have significant trauma histories that have not been worked through in therapy, or are prone to psychotic symptoms. As discussed in Chapter 1, we therefore need to be judicious in suggesting more intensive practice.

• *Is the meditation center reputable?* Obviously, we wouldn't want to encourage patients to practice with a particular teacher or at a particular center unless we were confident they would be treated with respect, sensitivity, and integrity. So before making a referral to a meditation center, it's a good idea to investigate the center's reputation, either by consulting with trusted colleagues or by going there ourselves. (The latter can lead to other potential problems, which we discuss shortly.)

Different Types of Centers

There are many places where one can learn and practice meditation. Some have roots in Christian, Jewish, Islamic, Yogic, and other religious traditions, whereas others are secular. Any of these might be best suited to our cultural background or that of our patients. But as previously discussed, most of the practices in this book, and all of the mindfulness-based clinical programs described earlier, have Buddhist roots. This is not just a coincidence—Buddhist traditions have created a remarkably nuanced body of teachings describing how meditation practices and techniques can be used to awaken the mind and heart.

Buddhist meditation centers typically emphasize one of three broad schools of practice. Because Western psychotherapists may be unfamiliar with these, a brief overview may be helpful. Determining which type of practice might be most suited for us, and potentially for our patients, depends on a combination of cultural affinity, learning style, and geographic convenience.

The vipassana, or insight meditation tradition, has arguably had the greatest influence on mindfulness-based practices that are currently being integrated with Western psychotherapy. *Vipassana* is usually translated as "seeing things as they are." Through this practice, we come to see things as they are by continually bringing our attention back to our bare experience instead of getting lost in the various interpretations and delusions our minds tend to create. Instructions in vipassana centers are usually laid out in a step-by-step fashion. Most of these centers have a Western cultural atmosphere. This is a form of practice most often seen in Southeast Asia.

Zen centers also teach mindfulness practice. Some provide step-by-step instructions similar to those we have described, whereas others suggest forms of meditation practice, such as *just sitting*, which doesn't focus on a particular object of attention, or koan practice, which asks students to solve a riddle that has no logical answer (to help interrupt discursive thinking). Their atmosphere may reflect their origins in Japanese, Korean, Chinese, or Vietnamese culture.

Tibetan Buddhist centers teach mindfulness practice along with other forms of meditation that may involve visualization of images, recitation of mantras, *tonglen* (giving and taking) practice, or prostrations (bowing). Their atmosphere often reflects their origin in Tibetan culture.

Residential versus Nonresidential Centers

Some meditation centers offer overnight accommodations for those interested in an extended stay. Others simply offer instruction and a quiet place to practice.

Nonresidential centers tend to be located in cities and other more populated areas. While they can't provide the intensity of a residential retreat, they do offer several advantages that aren't available at most residential centers: They're usually easier to get to. They provide a relatively easy, low-risk, low-cost way to test the waters for people who are skeptical, new to practice, and/or unsure about what kind of commitment they want to make. And finally, for those who attend regularly, they can offer a greater sense of community, as well as an opportunity to work more regularly with a teacher.

The biggest advantage of spending time at a residential retreat center is being free from the distractions of daily life and therefore able to steep oneself in meditation practice and reach deeper levels of concentration, mindfulness, and insight. But residential retreats are not easy. They require a considerable investment of time, and in most cases, money. And they can force us to look at all kinds of buried pain and inner conflicts, without the usual array of defenses we rely on to protect ourselves. So while they can be extremely valuable, as discussed in Chapter 1, silent residential retreats are not for everyone, and are especially not suitable for our most vulnerable patients.

Maintaining Professional Boundaries

As we mentioned above, when we start bringing mindfulness exercises into psychotherapy, the boundary between mental health professional and meditation teacher can get fuzzy, for the practitioner as well as the patient. And this raises important clinical and ethical questions. At what point does our work stop being psychiatric treatment and start becoming spiritual guidance? Do we tell the patient that this transition might take place? And if so, when? At the initial meeting? Later in treatment? Furthermore, if we perceive that we have moved beyond the traditional territory of psychotherapy, are we bound by the same professional codes of conduct? Do we charge the same fees? Can we bill insurance?

Even if we believe the work we're doing is totally secular and evidence-based mental health treatment, are we obligated to inform our patients about the Buddhist and other spiritual teachings from which mindfulness practice is derived? Is sneaking them in via a "Trojan horse" a deceptive way to practice?

These are complex questions without simple answers, about which intelligent, ethical, well-meaning professionals are likely to disagree. By asking these questions, we hope to encourage dialogue and reflection among the community of mindfulness-oriented psychotherapists, and to begin a process that will lead to more thoughtful and meaningful policies and practices in the future. We invite you to become part of the process by discussing them with trusted colleagues and supervisors.

We'd like to close with a brief word about boundary issues that may arise if you and your patient end up practicing at the same meditation center. In some ways, this is not so different from attending the same church or working out at the same gym. As in these other settings, it is important not to engage in dual relationships. So if you practice regularly at a particular meditation center, you may choose not to recommend it to patients. On the other hand, keeping it to yourself could be seen as withholding a potentially valuable resource. Of course, if you do recommend a center where you practice, it's best to be clear about this from the beginning and discuss whether it would be a problem for your patient to run into you there. We know clinicians who strictly avoid putting themselves in these kinds of situations, and others who feel they're appropriate or even useful with certain patients. Here, too, there are no simple rules or guidelines, other than to put the interests of the patients first.

For More Information

For a list of mindfulness-based clinical programs, residential and nonresidential retreat centers, as well as books, audio programs, and websites that can help you and your patients deepen your meditation practice, see the Resources.

*   *   *

As you've probably sensed, we find the practices presented throughout this book to be enormously useful in both our personal and professional lives. We're happy to have had the opportunity to share them here, and hope that they will help enrich your life both inside and outside of the clinical hour as much as they have enriched ours.

May you have many mindful moments!

APPENDIX

Selecting Practices

This Appendix suggests ways that various practices might be used with different psychological disorders and clinical populations. The practices listed can be used individually or introduced in the sequences presented. Of course, every patient is unique—these are merely suggestions based on our experience in the laboratory of the clinical hour. Please feel free to adapt them to suit the needs of particular individuals.

We typically introduce practices within sessions, practice with patients during the clinical hour, and then invite patients to try practicing at home. As mentioned earlier, recording meditation instructions in your own voice and giving them to your patient to use can add the support of the therapeutic alliance to your patient's meditation practice. If you prefer, you can also direct patients to the online reproducible handouts and audio recordings of selected practices available without charge at *www.sittingtogether.com*.

We have also highlighted in this Appendix practices designed to address the needs of the therapist, and have included a number of variations on practices presented previously that may be helpful in responding to particular therapeutic challenges.

PRACTICES FOR PARTICULAR DISORDERS

Addictive Disorders

- *Being Present* (page 140), an easily accessible way to introduce mindful awareness.
- *Standing Meditation* (page 142) to help ground and stabilize.
- *Finding the Breath* (page 73) to anchor awareness and lay a foundation for beginning again.
- *Touch Points* (page 70) with an optional focus on *Hands* (see page 204 in Additional Practices) to observe the urge to grasp the desired object.
- *Riding the Wave* (page 125) to tolerate the intensity of cravings.
- *Labeling Emotions* (page 94) to gain perspective and understanding.
- *Offering Loving-Kindness to Oneself* (page 103) to help soothe the self-criticism that often accompanies addiction.
- *Anchor at the Bottom of a Stormy Sea* (page 127), an "industrial-strength" practice that is helpful after a binge or during waves of particularly challenging emotion.
- *Compassionate Being* (page 112), for difficult times when isolation and self-hatred predominate.

Anxiety Disorders

- *Simply Listening* (page 68) to allow anxiety to come and go, just as sounds come and go.
- *Touch Points* (page 70) to find safety in the body and help tolerate strong sensations.
- *Body Sweep* (page 87) to use when physical symptoms of anxiety are intense.
- *Walking Meditation* (page 84) to use when feeling agitated and having difficulty sitting still. (See also *Walking in the World*, page 207, in Additional Practices.)
- *Thoughts Are Only Passing By* (see page 209 in Additional Practices) to help increase present-moment awareness.
- *Awareness of Emotions in the Body* (page 92) to increase capacity to be with anxiety.
- *Finding the Pattern* (page 97) to inquire into the habits of mind that may underlie anxiety.

- *Offering Loving-Kindness to Oneself* (page 103) when anxiety is accompanied by self-judgment and self-criticism. The phrases *May I be safe and protected* and *May I be at ease* can be particularly helpful.
- *Compassionate Body Scan* (page 105) to open to anxiety and develop compassion.
- *Mountain Meditation* (page 122) to develop equanimity around anxiety.

Depressive Disorders

- *Simply Listening* (page 68) to let depressive thoughts come and go.
- *Cradling the Breath* (page 76) to provide comfort in the midst of sadness or depression.
- *Walking Meditation* (page 84) to bring attention back to the experience of the present. Some meditation teachers also use *Silly Walking* (see page 208 in Additional Practices) to shift the mind away from preoccupation with ourselves and our problems.
- *Thoughts Are Only Passing By* (see page 209 in Additional Practices) to soften the pull of ruminative thoughts and increase present-moment awareness.
- *Awareness of Emotions in the Body* (page 92) to bring emotions that haven't been acknowledged into awareness.
- *Labeling Emotions* (page 94). Name them to tame them.
- *Finding the Pattern* (page 97) to see the pattern underlying depressive thoughts and feelings and how they link to behavior.
- *Compassionate Body Scan* (page 105) to reconnect with the body and bring compassionate attention to unpleasant thoughts, feelings, and physical sensations.
- *Compassionate Being* (page 112) when feeling isolated, overwhelmed, or in the depths of despair.
- *Connecting with the Suffering of Others* (page 117) to increase connection with others during times of intense pain and suffering.
- *Mountain Meditation* (page 122) to anchor attention in the ever-changing nature of life.
- *Anchor at the Bottom of a Stormy Sea* (page 127) to find safety below the waves of depressive thoughts and emotions.
- *Accepting the Challenge* (page 134) to get a different perspective on difficult circumstances.

- *Lotus Growing in a Murky Pond* (see page 205 in Additional Practices) to bring new understanding and meaning to depression.
- *Meditation with Light* (see page 206 in Additional Practices) to bring "light" to difficult times.

Eating Disorders

- *Touch Points* (page 70) to be with strong desires to binge, purge, or restrict. The variation *Hands* (see page 204 in Additional Practices) can also bring attention to these impulses.
- *Finding the Breath* (page 73) to develop a safe anchor in the body and learn that it is OK to begin again.
- *Awareness of Sensation* (page 89) to increase awareness of sensations that may precede binging or restricting.
- *Compassionate Eating* (page 108) to practice eating mindfully and with compassion for one's body.
- *Riding the Wave* (page 125) for times when cravings are hard to tolerate.
- *Forgiveness: Letting Go of Poison* (page 132) to forgive oneself after bingeing.

Physical Pain

- *Touch Points* (page 70) to find ease in the body and relax into the pain.
- *Finding the Breath* (page 73) to allow pain to arise and fall away, just like the breath.
- *Awareness of Sensation* (page 89) to bring awareness to the sensations of the pain and increase the capacity to bear it.
- *Being with Discomfort* (page 49) to open to, rather than resist, unpleasant sensations.
- *Compassionate Body Scan* (page 105) to be with unpleasant sensations and bring compassion to ourselves because we are in pain.
- *Thoughts Are Only Passing By* (see page 209 in Additional Practices) to heighten awareness of the relationship between thoughts about pain and the sensations themselves.
- *Mountain Meditation* (page 122) to find stability and balance within the pain.
- *Walking in the World* (see page 207 in Additional Practices) to anchor the attention in the world outside painful sensations.

- *Riding the Wave* (page 125) when feeling desperate about or overwhelmed by the pain.

Sleep Disorders

- *Touch Points* (page 70) with a focus on the parts of the body that are touching the bed.
- *Finding the Breath* (page 73) and *Cradling the Breath* (page 76) to be with regrets and worry that may arise in the middle of the night.
- *Letting Go of the Story* (page 77) if past events are making sleep difficult.
- *Awareness of Sensation* (page 89) if bodily discomfort is disrupting sleep.
- *Being with Discomfort* (page 49) to open to, rather than resist, unpleasant sensations.
- *Labeling Emotions* (page 94) to identify and let go of emotions and thoughts.
- *Finding the Pattern* (page 97) to bring awareness of how sensations, thoughts, and emotions combine to keep the mind awake.
- *Compassionate Body Scan* (page 105) to cultivate compassion for any suffering that may be arising.
- *Compassionate Being* (page 112) when self-compassion is elusive.
- *Accepting the Challenge* (page 134) when ruminating about a situation and wanting to see it in a new way.
- *All Things Must Pass* (page 136) when resistance to illness, aging, and death is keeping us awake.

Trauma

- *Simply Listening* (page 68) to anchor in present-moment awareness.
- *Touch Points* (page 70) to establish an experience of safety in the body.
- *Cradling the Breath* (page 76) to bring comfort and soothe oneself.
- *Letting Go of the Story* (page 77) to work with the rumination that often accompanies posttraumatic stress disorder.
- *Walking Meditation* (page 84) as well as *Walking in the World* (see page 207 in Additional Practices) to stay present when feeling overwhelmed.
- *Mini-Mindfulness Break* (page 39) when feeling flooded by memories, thoughts, or feelings.

- *Awareness of Emotions in the Body* (page 92) to bring attention to unacknowledged emotions.
- *Labeling Emotions* (page 94). Name them to tame them.
- *Offering Loving-Kindness to Oneself* (page 103) to soothe a self-critical inner dialogue.
- *Bringing Compassion into Daily Life* (page 110) because it is often easier to send compassion to others.
- *Compassionate Being* (page 112) for especially difficult, self-critical times.
- *Connecting with the Suffering of Others* (page 117) to ease isolation and connect with others.
- *Mountain Meditation* (page 122) to cultivate acceptance of traumatic events.
- *Anchor at the Bottom of a Stormy Sea* (page 127) to find stability amid the storms of life.
- *Accepting the Challenge* (page 134) to recognize unacknowledged strengths.

PRACTICES FOR PARTICULAR POPULATIONS

Children and Adolescents

- *Being Present* (page 140), an easily accessible way to introduce mindful awareness.
- *Standing Meditation* (page 142) to help ground and develop steadiness.
- *Simply Listening* (page 68) to help develop attention. Chris Willard (2010) suggests having children count the number of different sounds they hear.
- *Silly Walking* (see page 208 in Additional Practices). A playful variation on walking meditation especially suited to children.
- *Soles of the Feet* (see page 209 in Additional Practices) to bring attention back to the sensory experience in the present.
- *Thoughts Are Only Passing By* (see page 209 in Additional Practices). Children tend to particularly enjoy the cloud and wave practices.
- *Labeling Emotions* (page 94). Name them to tame them—at any age.
- *Mind That Sparkles* (see page 207 in Additional Practices), a fun way to illustrate the swirling nature of our thoughts and feelings.

- *Offering Loving-Kindness to Oneself* (page 103) to comfort when circumstances are difficult.

- *Opening to Kindness* (page 146) to strengthen the capacity to be kind to oneself.

- *Bringing Compassion into Daily Life* (page 110), an active practice often used in classrooms.

- *Riding the Wave* (page 125) to be with strong feelings and urges.

Couples and Families

- *Pausing* (page 37) to help ground and take some "time-in" during a disagreement.

- *Mini-Mindfulness Break* (page 39) to take a minute to ground and gain perspective.

- *Simply Listening* (page 68; see also *Listening to Another*, page 204 in Additional Practices) to help partners listen to each other.

- *Breathing Together* (page 60) to deepen the connection between partners or family members.

- *What Brings You Away?* (page 47) to help bring awareness to ways we disconnect from others.

- *Letting Go of the Story* (page 77) to allow obsessive thoughts and destructive emotions to arise and fall away.

- *Labeling Emotions* (page 94) to increase awareness of the feelings that are being triggered in the relationship.

- *Seeing with Loving Eyes* (see page 208 in Additional Practices) to help see relationships in a new light.

- *Offering Loving-Kindness to Oneself* (page 103) to bring kindness to oneself during relationship challenges.

- *Working with a Difficult Person* (page 114) to bring compassion and understanding to a difficult relationship.

- *Sympathetic Joy* (page 129) to cultivate pleasure in another's good fortune.

- *Forgiveness: Letting Go of Poison* (page 132) if possible and only if ready.

- *Anchor at the Bottom of a Stormy Sea* (page 127) to find some balance during challenging times.

- *Accepting the Challenge* (page 134) for use during holidays, weddings, and divorces, to help accept things as they are.

PRACTICES FOR THE CLINICIAN

In addition to the meditations suggested in Chapters 2 and 3, we've found
the following ones helpful to foster attunement, recover equilibrium
after a difficult session, or recharge when feeling stressed or burnt out.

- *Working with a Difficult Person* (page 114) when feeling angry or losing
  sleep about a patient.
- *Compassionate Being* (page 112) when feeling that we need additional
  support and compassion.
- *Anchor at the Bottom of a Stormy Sea* (page 127) to help accept the feelings that arise after difficult interactions, including patient self-harm.
- *Four-Elements Meditation* (see page 203 in Additional Practices) to use
  when feeling upset, depleted, or distraught after a session.
- *Listening to Another* (see page 204 in Additional Practices) to help listen
  to patients deeply.
- *Loving-Kindness for Clinicians* (see page 205 in Additional Practices) to
  increase feelings of loving-kindness and self-compassion.

ADDITIONAL PRACTICES

These are variations on practices presented earlier that may suit the
needs of particular people or situations. Before beginning these exercises, start by finding your seat and adopting a posture of dignity.
Spend a few moments settling into your anchor (touch points, breath,
or sound) and being present with your experience.

This first meditation is inspired by the Tibetan practice of *tonglen* (giving and receiving). In the traditional exercise, you breathe in
the pain and suffering of others and breathe out compassion. We have
found, however, that for many patients, breathing in more pain is overwhelming. In this variation, you breathe in compassion and breathe out
compassion. Check in with the patient to assess how it is going. As with
any practice, keep it short, especially when you first introduce it, and
feel free to return to sounds, the breath, or awareness of the body if the
patient needs more grounding.

COMPASSION IN THE MOMENT

- Start by sitting comfortably, taking a few breaths to anchor yourself.
- Bring your awareness into your body and notice where you

feel discomfort or distress. Notice any difficult emotions that might be present. If a particular person is associated with this discomfort, note that as well.

- Inhale deeply, bringing compassion into your body and to the places where you are experiencing stress, pain, or unpleasant emotions.

- As you exhale, send compassion to the person associated with the discomfort, to others who might experience similar difficulty, or to all beings.

- Breathe compassion in and out, finding a rhythm that feels comfortable. You may want to imagine that you are being rocked and soothed by your breath.

- Visualize filling every cell of your body with compassion, inhaling it for yourself, exhaling it for others.

This practice is adapted from Morgan, Morgan, and Germer (2013). Copyright 2013 by The Guilford Press. Adapted by permission.

The *Four-Elements Meditation* can help us find balance after a difficult interaction or an upsetting event. It is especially useful after a challenging session:

FOUR-ELEMENTS MEDITATION

- *Earth.* Breathe in and out through your nose for five to ten breaths. Visualize a magnificent mountain while you are breathing. Feel yourself becoming grounded and rooted in the earth.

- *Water.* Breathe in through the nose and out through the mouth for five to ten breaths. Imagine a waterfall flowing through and cleansing your body and refreshing your spirit. Let go of any tightness or tension that you might be holding.

- *Fire.* Breathe in through your mouth and out through your nose for five to ten breaths. Visualize the warmth and energy of a gentle fire.

- *Air.* Breathe in through your mouth and out through your mouth five to ten times. Visualize the spaciousness and openness of the sky. See if you can bring this lightness to your body and mind. Rest here for a few moments.

Inspired by the teaching of Pir Vilayat Inayat Khan.

This next practice is helpful with entrenched addictive disorders, as it can bring increased awareness to the urge to grasp a desired object. It is a variation on the practice of *Touch Points* and is another way to increase our capacity to tolerate strong or overwhelming desires.

HANDS

- Let your hands rest in your lap. Bring your awareness to them, feeling them from the inside (the muscles and bones) to the outside (the skin and nails).

- Bring your attention to any sensations that you notice either inside your hands or where they touch your skin or your clothing. Allow your hands to settle into the stillness, not grasping anything, not pushing away anything.

- Become curious about what happens in your body when you allow your hands to rest. Bring your awareness to any sensations, thoughts, and feelings that you notice. Allow any desires (e.g., for food, a substance, entertainment) to arise and pass away.

- Keep returning your attention to your hands, feeling any and all sensations that arise. Let your hands be just as they are in this moment.

The following practice can increase our ability to listen to painful and upsetting content. We have found it helpful when listening to stories of extreme trauma and abuse or for any time that a clinician feels helpless.

LISTENING TO ANOTHER

- As you sit and listen to another person, see if you can do so with "beginner's mind." Listen with your entire being, as if you have never heard this person speak before. Bring all your interest and curiosity.

- See if you can listen without judgment or prejudice. Notice any agenda you might have. You do not have to change or fix this person. Simply be present, attuned to subtle qualities of voice and intonation.

- Become aware of moments where there might be hidden sadness, anger, or another emotion behind the words.

- If you find yourself becoming distracted, notice any resistance and return your attention to fully listening.

  Inspired by the following invocation taught at Cambridge Insight Meditation Society: "We will sit and listen without judging or reacting. We will sit and listen in order to understand. We will practice listening so attentively that we will be able to hear what is being said as well as what is being left unsaid. For we know that just by listening deeply we already alleviate a great deal of pain and suffering."

This next practice can bring new perspective and understanding to a depressive episode. We have used it to increase the capacity to be with painful feelings in treatment-resistant depression.

LOTUS GROWING IN A MURKY POND

- Begin with an image of a beautiful lotus floating in the center of a pond. Imagine that you can follow its long stem to where the plant is anchored in the mud and decay at the bottom. The flower is not separate from the dark and murky waters but is nourished by and takes its life and nutrients from them.

- Try sitting upright in your experience of depression and suffering. The lotus offers us a lesson in metabolizing the darkness.

- What depth, sustenance, or richness can you find in your challenging experience?

  Inspired by a meditation taught by Trudy Goodman.

These additional loving-kindness phrases can help us refocus and recharge during periods of stress. They can also help us find balance and increase attunement with demanding or difficult patients.

LOVING-KINDNESS FOR CLINICIANS

- May I be able to care for and nurture myself so I can attend to the needs of others with generosity, balance, and presence.

- May I develop equanimity and let go of expectations of healing or curing others.

- May I see this person with a freshness of mind and an openness of heart.

- While I care about your pain and suffering, I cannot make choices for you or control your life.
- May I accept the limitations of others with warmth and compassion, and may I accept my own limits with the same kindness.
- May I see you, hear you, and know you in your wholeness and beauty—not just in your suffering and pain.
- May I see the goodness, intelligence, and vulnerability in this person.
- May I let this moment be as it is, not as I want it to be.

Inspired by Sharon Salzberg (2011).

The following practice can help bring "light" to difficult situations. It is also a meditation that can be used to begin the day, before greeting patients, or when we need to refresh during the day.

MEDITATION WITH LIGHT

- Imagine that you are sitting and watching a spectacular sunrise with a wide spectrum of soft, luminous colors.
- As the sun rises over the horizon, feel it gently warming and illuminating your body; at first the face, then the neck, chest, arms, torso, pelvis, legs, and feet.
- If it feels comfortable, allow the light to enter your body, filling it with a golden glow. Feel the light touching the dark places within yourself, any place where you hold pain or sorrow.
- Let the light fill your entire body, touching your bones, your muscles, your internal organs, veins, arteries—every cell of your body. Imagine your entire body sparkling and radiating light.
- Rest in this light; let yourself become "a lamp unto yourself."

Inspired by the teaching of Pir Vilayat Inayat Khan.

Our minds can be like blizzards in a snow globe. When we're upset, our thoughts and feelings swirl around and around, just like a big storm. This next exercise can help us to see what it is like to let things clear—and when done with a real snow globe, can be an accessible illustration for children.

MIND THAT SPARKLES

- Try to feel three breaths, letting your body and mind slow down a little. See if you can watch one thought, like a storm cloud, rise and fall away. When our mind and body are really agitated, it is hard to see clearly, just like in a shaken snow globe. For just a minute or two, practice sitting still and settling into the quiet.

- If you like, make your own snow globe, filling a glass jar with water and glitter. Shake it up and then watch the sparkles settle and fall to the bottom of the jar. See what happens if you stick a finger in the jar and try to force it down. Does it make the process go faster?

- As the glitter clears, tune into your breath and your body and see what you notice.

Inspired by Chris Willard (2010).

The following practice, a variation on *Walking Meditation,* is helpful when one is agitated or having difficulty sitting still. We have used it with patients who feel confined in a small office (and feel safer being outside). It can also help anchor the attention in the world outside of painful physical sensations or emotions.

WALKING IN THE WORLD

- Take a few minutes and go outside. Bring your attention to the sky, no matter what the weather.

- Spend a moment watching the clouds, feeling the wind, whether it is warm or cold, wet or dry.

- Look up at the trees; notice the colors of the leaves, their texture, the way that the light comes through them.

- Listen: Do you hear birds singing? Dogs barking? Children playing?

- As you begin to walk, notice grass or flowers that may be growing, and pay attention to their colors and form. Look at the ground, becoming aware of insects, puddles, even the rainbows that sometimes form when oil mixes with water.

- See the world with a child's eyes, as if it is all new. If you live in a city, bring attention to the noise of traffic, cars, and buses passing by, people rushing down the street—the colors, sounds, smells.

- If you find yourself preoccupied with pain, anxiety, or ruminative thoughts, note this and then add, "and the leaves are golden," or "and the traffic is passing by."

When a baby is born, we fall in love. When we hold an adorable puppy, we see with loving eyes. But over time, after injuries and disappointments, our glance can become harsh, angry, and critical. We often focus on what we believe is wrong with another. This next practice can be especially helpful when our pain has caused us to become hardened.

SEEING WITH LOVING EYES

- Experiment with looking at people with kind and loving eyes. As you do, bring awareness to any tension or tightness around your eyes; invite, but don't force, your eyes to soften.
- Bring attention to any subtle shifts in the face, body, heart, and mind. Notice any stories that come to mind or any resistance that arises; allow it to rise and fall away without getting caught in the narrative.
- See what happens when you soften your gaze: Look at your partner, your child, a colleague with kind and loving eyes. It is usually not a one-way experience. How we look at others often colors the way they look at us, and in turn the way we see ourselves.

Many meditation teachers teach this practice; this version was inspired by Bays (2011).

The following practice is a variation on Monty Python's "Ministry of Silly Walks," which can be found on YouTube *www.youtube.com/watch?v=iV2ViNJFZC8*. It is taught by meditation and yoga teachers as a fun way to inhabit the body. And it's a great practice for children. We have also found that some patients (and therapists) suffering from anxiety, depression, and trauma can benefit from this practice.

SILLY WALKING

- Take a few minutes to do a "silly walk." This can mean taking huge steps, walking sideways like a crab, or walking backward. You can even skip or hop if you like.

- Try to fully inhabit your body as you walk, noticing sensations. Don't worry about how you look—this exercise is about having fun and learning to be in your body.
- Enjoy!

This practice is a quick way to help patients (and their therapists) become more grounded, literally, and is especially useful when working with aggressive or impulsive behavior. With children, it can be an effective way to begin to cultivate attention. It can be done either standing or sitting.

SOLES OF THE FEET

- Start by rocking back and forth, from the heels to the toes, and then side to side. Wiggle your toes.
- If you like, raise one foot and then the other, as if you are marching.
- Feel your feet resting firmly on the ground. Notice all of the different sensations. Feel the soles of your feet.
- If you like, imagine that there are roots underneath each foot, anchoring and grounding you. Let yourself feel connected to the earth.
- If you get distracted, simply return to feeling the soles of your feet.

This next practice increases awareness of the present moment. It is appealing to children, but adults also appreciate its focus on images of the natural world. It can be especially powerful when done outside, lying down and watching the sky.

THOUGHTS ARE ONLY PASSING BY

- Once you feel grounded and centered, bring your attention to your thoughts. Watch the thoughts as they arise, imagining them as clouds passing through the sky. Some are fluffy cumulus, others are dark and stormy. Sometimes there are few clouds, other times the sky is totally clouded over.
- Let them all pass by. Know that you are not the thoughts. See if you can imagine yourself as the vast and spacious sky that is holding all this constantly changing weather.

- (A variation is to visualize that you are at a beach where the sand and water meet. Let yourself rest there for a minute watching the waves come and go. Inhale. Notice the smell, the sounds, the rhythm of the ocean. Take a stick or a rock and write down any anxious or ruminative thoughts in the wet sand. Watch as a wave comes and the words disappear into the wet sand.)
- Let the clouds be clouds (or the waves be waves). As Zen masters say, thoughts are "real but not true." Let the thoughts pass by and disappear without clinging to them.

The following practice can be comforting in the aftermath of traumatic events, such as mass shootings and bombings, as well as natural disasters, such as earthquakes, severe storms, and floods.

SHELTER IN PLACE

- Take a few deep breaths and come into the present moment, knowing that you are sitting. You can keep your eyes either open or closed.
- Bring to mind those who were harmed, those who responded, those who witnessed, both in person and through the media, all those who were and perhaps still are frightened.
- Breathe in love and compassion, breathe out love and compassion. Be sure to include yourself, especially on the inbreath.
- For those who were wounded, in whatever way, breathe with them. Breathe in courage, strength, dignity, and compassion; breathe out courage, strength, dignity, and compassion.
- For the friends and families, for the caretakers, for all who are helping others hold the pain, shock, and terror, breathe in love and compassion; breathe out love and compassion.
- For all communities, all countries, where there have been tragedies and disasters, breathe in love and compassion, breathe out love and compassion.
- If you meet resistance, anger, fear, or grief, allow it to be. Breathe in love and compassion, breathe out love, compassion, spaciousness, and ease.
- Try repeating these, or similar phrases silently:

- *May all your sorrows be eased, May your hearts and bodies be soothed and healed.*
- *May all beings be safe and protected, May all be free from suffering, May all beings live in wisdom and compassion.*

Inspired by a dharma talk given by Jack Kornfield (2013).

As mentioned in Chapter 8, many patients find it helpful to carry reminders of practice principles written on flash cards. The following instructions present one way to introduce these.

FLASH CARDS

Copy some of your favorite phrases from the list below onto small cards you can carry with you or post somewhere in your home, car, or workplace. Feel free to modify them or add your own phrases at the end of the list. Refer to them whenever you need encouragement, support, or a reminder to be mindful.

1. *May I be safe and protected from inner and outer harm.*
2. *May I meet this moment fully, may I meet it as a friend.*
3. *This is a moment of pain. Every human being experiences pain. Life is often difficult. Let me be kind to myself.*
4. *My sweet body, you are doing the best you can.*
5. *If it isn't happening now, it isn't happening.*
6. *That was then, this is now.*
7. *Just the breath, nothing else.*
8. *Can I create space for this?*
9. *A thought that I am . . . (anxious/unlovable/a loser, etc.).*
10. *It's OK to begin again.*
11. *May I accept things just as they are.*
12. *May I love myself completely, just the way I am.*

13. _____

14. _____

15. _____

Resources

Throughout this book, we have drawn upon practices presented by many different teachers from many different traditions, both spiritual and secular. To learn more about some of their approaches to meditation and mindfulness practice, you may wish to consult the books and recordings listed below.

For those who would like to deepen their practice, we've also included an extensive but by no means comprehensive listing of meditation centers worldwide, as well as contact information for organizations that offer more intensive mindfulness training in clinical settings.

BOOKS ABOUT MINDFULNESS MEDITATION

Books by Meditation and Spiritual Teachers

The following are a few of the books that have been most influential in our own learning, or which we recommend most frequently to patients and colleagues interested in developing their mindfulness practice.

Brach, T. (2003). *Radical acceptance: Embracing your life with the heart of a Buddha.* New York: Bantam/Dell.

Chodron, P. (1997). *When things fall apart: Heart advice for difficult times.* Boston: Shambhala.

Chodron, P. (2009). *Taking the leap: Freeing ourselves from old habits and fears.* Boston: Shambhala.

Dalai Lama. (2001). *An open heart: Practicing compassion in everyday life.* New York: Little, Brown.

Dalai Lama, & Cutler, H. (1998). *The art of happiness: A handbook for living.* New York: Riverhead Books.

Goldstein, J. (1993) *Insight meditation: The practice of freedom.* Boston: Shambhala.

Goldstein, J., & Kornfield, J. (1987). *Seeking the heart of wisdom.* Boston: Shambhala.

Gunaratana, B. (2002). *Mindfulness in plain English.* Somerville, MA: Wisdom.

Hanh, T. N. (1976). *The miracle of mindfulness.* Boston: Beacon Press.

Hanh, T. N. (1991). *Peace in every step: The path of mindfulness in everyday life.* New York: Bantam.

Helminski, K. E. (1992). *Living presence: A Sufi way to mindfulness and the essential self.* New York: Tarcher/Perigree Books.

Kabat-Zinn, J. (1994). *Wherever you go there you are: Mindfulness meditation in everyday life.* New York: Hyperion.

Keating, T. (2006). *Open mind, open heart: The contemplative dimension of the Gospel.* New York: Continuum International Group.

Kornfield, J. (1993). *A path with heart: A guide through the perils and promises of spiritual life.* New York: Bantam.

Kornfield, J. (2008). *The wise heart: A guide to the universal teachings of Buddhist psychology.* New York: Bantam.

Lama Surya Das. (1998). *Awakening the Buddha within: Tibetan wisdom for the western world.* New York: Doubleday.

Lew, A. (2005). *Be still and get going: A Jewish meditation practice for real life.* Boston: Little, Brown.

Pennington, M. B. (1982). *Centering prayer: Renewing an ancient Christian prayer form.* Garden City, NY: Image Books.

Rosenberg, L. (2004). *Breath by breath: The liberating practice of insight meditation.* Boston: Shambhala.

Salzberg, S. (1995). *Lovingkindness: The revolutionary art of happiness.* Boston: Shambhala.

Salzberg, S. (2011). *Real happiness: The power of meditation.* New York: Workman.

Suzuki, S. (1973*). Zen mind, beginner's mind.* New York: Weatherhill.

Clinically Oriented Books

The following are a few of the clinical resources we recommend most frequently to our patients and colleagues:

Bien, T. (2006). *Mindful therapy: A guide for therapists and helping professionals.* Boston: Wisdom Publications.

Brantley, J. (2003). *Calming your anxious mind.* Oakland, CA: New Harbinger.

Forsyth, J., & Eifert, G. (2008). *The mindfulness and acceptance workbook for anxiety.* Oakland, CA: New Harbinger.

Germer, C. K. (2009). *The mindful path to self-compassion: Freeing yourself from destructive thoughts and emotions.* New York: Guilford Press.

Germer, C. K., & Siegel, R. D. (Eds.). (2012). *Wisdom and compassion in psychotherapy: Deepening mindfulness in clinical practice.* New York: Guilford Press.

Germer, C. K., Siegel, R. D., & Fulton, P. R. (Eds.). (2013). *Mindfulness and psychotherapy* (2nd ed.). New York: Guilford Press.

Hayes, S., & Smith, S. (2005). *Get out of your mind and into your life: The new acceptance and commitment therapy.* Oakland, CA: New Harbinger.

Kabat-Zinn, J. (1990). *Full catastrophe living: Using the wisdom of your body and mind to face stress, pain, and illness.* New York: Dell.

Kabat-Zinn, J. (2005). *Coming to our senses: Healing ourselves and the world through mindfulness.* New York: Hyperion.

Linehan, M. M. (1993). *Skills training manual for treating borderline personality disorder.* New York: Guilford Press.

Neff, K. D. (2011). *Self-compassion: Stop beating yourself up and leave insecurity behind.* New York: William Morrow.

Orsillo, S. M., & Roemer, L. (2011). *The mindful way through anxiety: Break free from chronic worry and redeem your life.* New York: Guilford Press.

Peltz, L. (2013). *The mindful path to addiction recovery: A practical guide to regaining control over your life.* Boston: Shambhala.

Segal, Z. V., Williams, J. M. G., & Teasdale, J. D. (2012). *Mindfulness-based cognitive therapy for depression (2nd ed.).* New York: Guilford Press.

Siegel, D. J. (2010). *The mindful therapist: A clinician's guide to mindsight and neural integration.* New York: W. W. Norton.

Siegel, R. D. (2010). *The mindfulness solution: Everyday practices for everyday problems.* New York: Guilford Press.

Stahl, B., & Goldstein, E. (2010). *A mindfulness-based stress reduction workbook.* Oakland, CA: New Harbinger.

Strosahl, K., & Robinson, P. (2008). *The mindfulness and acceptance workbook for depression.* Oakland, CA: New Harbinger.

Williams, J. M. G., Teasdale, J. D., Segal, Z. V., & Kabat-Zinn, J. (2007). *The mindful way through depression: Freeing yourself from chronic unhappiness.* New York: Guilford Press.

RECORDINGS

Free downloads of talks from insight meditation retreats: *www.dharmaseed.org*

General recordings from mindfulness meditation teachers: *www.soundstrue.com*

Recordings and Teaching Schedules of Selected Meditation Teachers

Vipassana (Insight Meditation) Tradition

Tara Brach: *www.tarabrach.com*

Jack Kornfield: *www.jackkornfield.com*

Sharon Salzberg: *www.sharonsalzberg.com*

Zen Tradition

Thich Nhat Hanh: *www.iamhome.org*, *www.plumvillage.org*

Tibetan Buddhist Tradition

Pema Chödrön: *www.shambhala.org/teachers/pema*

Dalai Lama: *www.dalailama.com*

Lama Surya Das: *www.dzogchen.org*

Christian Tradition (Contemplative or Centering Prayer)

Father William Menninger: *www.contemplativeprayer.net*

MEDITATION CENTERS

United States

Vipassana (Insight Meditation) Tradition

Barre Center for Buddhist Studies
149 Lockwood Road
Barre, MA 01005
www.dharma.org/bcbs

Bhavana Society
Route 1, Box 218-3
High View, WV 26808
www.bhavanasociety.org

Cambridge Insight Meditation Center
331 Broadway
Cambridge, MA 02139
www.cambridgeinsight.org

InsightLA
2633 Lincoln Boulevard, #206
Santa Monica, CA 90405–2005
www.insightla.org

Insight Meditation Community of Washington
PO Box 3
Cabin John, MD 20818
www.imcw.org

Insight Meditation Society
1230 Pleasant Street
Barre, MA 01005
www.dharma.org

Metta Forest Monastery
PO Box 1419
Valley Center, CA 92082
www.watmetta.org

Mid America Dharma
455 East 80th Terrace
Kansas City, MO 64131
www.midamericadharma.org

New York Insight Meditation Center
28 West 27th Street, 10th floor
New York, NY 10001
www.nyimc.org

Spirit Rock Meditation Center
PO Box 909
Woodacre, CA 94973
www.spiritrock.org

Zen Tradition

Blue Cliff Monastery
3 Mindfulness Road
Pine Bush, NY 12566
www.bluecliffmonastery.org

Boundless Way Zen
297 Lowell Avenue
Newton, MA 02460-1826
www.boundlesswayzen.org

Cambridge Zen Center
199 Auburn Street
Cambridge, MA 02139
www.cambridgezen.com

Deer Park Monastery
2499 Melru Lane
Escondido, CA 92026
www.deerparkmonastery.org

San Francisco Zen Center
300 Page Street
San Francisco, CA 94102
www.sfzc.org

Upaya Zen Center
1404 Cerro Gordo Road
Santa Fe, NM 87501
www.upaya.org

Village Zendo
588 Broadway, Suite 1108
New York, NY 10012-5238
www.villagezendo.org

Zen Center of San Diego
2047 Feldspar Street
San Diego, CA 92109-3551
www.zencentersandiego.org

Zen Mountain Monastery
PO Box 197
Mt. Tremper, NY 12457
www.mro.org/zmm

Tibetan Buddhist Tradition

Dzogchen Center
www.dzogchen.org

Naropa University
2130 Arapahoe Avenue
Boulder, CO 80302
www.naropa.edu

Shambhala Mountain Center
4921 Country Road 68C
Red Feather Lakes, CO 80545
www.shambhalamountain.org

Tenzin Gyatso Institute
PO Box 239
Berne, NY 12023
www.tenzingyatsoinstitute.org

Insight Dialogue (Interpersonal Buddhist Meditation)

Metta Programs
PO Box 99172
Seattle, WA 98139
www.metta.org

Listing of additional Buddhist meditation centers and communities:

www.dharma.org/ims/mr_links.html

Jewish Traditions

(These vary in their degree of emphasis on mindfulness practice.)

Awakened Heart Project for Contemplative Judaism

www.awakenedheartproject.org

Institute for Jewish Spirituality
330 Seventh Avenue, Suite 1902
New York, NY 10001
www.ijs-online.org

Isabella Freedman Jewish Retreat Center
116 Johnson Road
Falls Village, CT 06031
www.isabellafreedman.org

Nishmat Hayyim
Jewish Meditation Collaborative of New England
1566 Beacon Street
Brookline, MA 02446
www.nishmathayyim.org

Christian Traditions (Contemplative or Centering Prayer)

Listing of programs throughout the United States and the world:
Contemplative Outreach
10 Park Place, 2nd Floor, Suite B
Butler, NJ 07405
www.contemplativeoutreach.org

Sufi Tradition

Sufi Order International
PO Box 480
New Lebanon, NY 12125
www.sufiorder.org

Canada

Gampo Abbey
Pleasant Bay, Cape Breton
Nova Scotia, BOE 2PO
Canada
www.gampoabbey.org

Listing of other Canadian meditation centers:

www.gosit.org/Canada.htm

Europe

Vipassana (Insight Meditation) Tradition

Gaia House
West Ogwell, Newton Abbot
Devon, TQ12 6EN
United Kingdom
www.gaiahouse.co.uk

Kalyana Centre
Glenahoe Castlegregory
Co Kerry
Ireland
www.kalyanacentre.com

Meditationszentrum Beatenberg Waldegg
CH–3803 Beatenberg
Switzerland
www.karuna.ch

Seminarhaus Engl
Engl 1
84339 Unterdietfurt
Bavaria
Germany
www.seminarhaus-engl.de

Listing of other European vipassana centers:

www.mahasi.eu

Zen Tradition

Plum Village Practice Center
13 Martineau
33580 Dieulivol
France
www.plumvillage.org

Tibetan Buddhist Tradition

Shambhala Europe
Kartäuserwall 20
50678 Köln
Germany
www.shambhala-europe.org

For Shambhala centers worldwide:

www.shambhala.org/centers

Sanctuary of Enlightened Action
Lerab Ling
34650 Roquerdonde
France
www.lerabling.org (see *www.rigpa.org* for related centers)

Australia and New Zealand

Vipassana (Insight Meditation) Tradition

Bodhinyanarama Monastery
17 Rakau Grove, Stokes Valley
Lower Hutt 5019
New Zealand
www.bodhinyanarama.net.nz

Santi Forest Monastery
Lot 6 Coalmines Road
Bundanoon, NSW, 2578
Australia
www.santifm.org

Listings of other Australian insight meditation centers:

www.bswa.org and *www.dharma.org.au*

Listing of other New Zealand insight meditation centers:

www.insightmeditation.org.nz

Zen Tradition

Listing of Zen centers in Australia:

http://iriz.hanazono.ac.jp/zen_centers/centers_data/australi.htm

Listing of Zen centers in New Zealand:

http://iriz.hanazono.ac.jp/zen_centers/centers_data/newzeal.htm

Tibetan Buddhist Tradition

Shambhala Meditation Centre Auckland
35 Scarborough Terrace
Auckland, New Zealand
www.auckland.shambhala.info

Worldwide

Listing of Buddhist meditation centers worldwide:

www.buddhanet.info/wbd

MINDFULNESS TRAINING IN CLINICAL SETTINGS

Mindfulness-Based Stress Reduction:
Center for Mindfulness in Medicine, Health Care, and Society
55 Lake Avenue North
Worcester, MA 01655
www.umassmed.edu/cfm

Mindfulness-Based Stress Reduction
and Mindfulness-Based Cognitive Therapy:
Centre for Mindfulness Research and Practice
Institute for Medical and Social Care Research
University of Wales
Bangor, LL57 1UT
United Kingdom
www.bangor.ac.uk/mindfulness

Acceptance and Commitment Therapy:

www.contextualpsychology.org/act

Dialectical Behavior Therapy:

www.behavioraltech.org

Mindfulness-Based Cognitive Therapy:

www.mbct.com

Mindfulness-Based Relapse Prevention:

www.depts.washington.edu/abrc/mbrp

Mindfulness-Based Eating Awareness Training:

www.tcme.org

The Institute for Meditation and Psychotherapy:

www.meditationandpsychotherapy.org

The Back Sense program for mindfulness-oriented treatment
of chronic pain:

www.backsense.org

Archives of the mindfulness and acceptance listserv
of the Association for Advancement of Behavior Therapy
(now the Association for Behavioral and Cognitive Therapies):

http://listserv.kent.edu/cgi-bin/wa.exe?INDEX

References

Armstrong, K. (2010). *Twelve steps to a compassionate life.* New York: Knopf.

Auerbach, H. H., & Johnson, M. (1977). Research on the therapist's level of experience. In A. S. Gurman & A. M. Razin (Eds.), *Effective psychotherapy: A handbook of research* (pp. 84–102). New York: Pergamon.

Bartlett, J. (1980). *Familiar quotations* (15th ed.). Boston: Little, Brown.

Batchelor, S. (1998). *Buddhism without beliefs: A contemporary guide to awakening.* New York: Riverhead Books.

Batchelor, S. (2010). *Confession of a Buddhist atheist.* New York, NY: Random House.

Bays, J. C. (2011). *How to train a wild elephant & other adventures in mindfulness.* Boston: Shambala.

Bien, T. (2006). *Mindful therapy: A guide for therapists and helping professionals.* Boston: Wisdom.

Boorstein, S. (2007). *Happiness is an inside job.* New York: Ballantine Books.

Boorstein, S. (2011a). *A path to happiness: A psychotherapist's guide to mindfulness.* Transcript of teleseminar session, National Institute for the Clinical Application of Behavioral Medicine.

Boorstein, S. (2011b, May 6). What we nurture [Audio podcast], In K. Tippett, *On being.* Retrieved from *www.onbeing.org/program/what-we-nurture/242/audio?embed=1.*

Bowen, S., Chawla, N., & Marlatt, G. A. (2011). *Mindfulness-based relapse prevention for addictive behaviors.* New York: Guilford Press.

Brach, T. (2003). *Radical acceptance: Embracing your life with the heart of a Buddha.* New York: Bantam Books.

Brach, T. (2011). *Meditation and psychotherapy* [Audio CD]. Boulder, CO: Sounds True.

Brach, T. (2012). *True refuge: Finding peace and freedom in our own awakened heart.* New York: Bantam Books.

Brach, T. (2013, March 30). *True refuge: Three gateways of emotional healing and spiritual freedom.* Workshop at the Cambridge Insight Meditation Center, Cambridge, MA.

Brewer, J. A. (2013). Breaking the addiction loop. In C. K. Germer, R. D. Siegel, & P. R. Fulton (Eds.), *Mindfulness and psychotherapy* (2nd ed.), pp. 225–238). New York: Guilford Press.

Briere, J. (2012). Working with trauma: Mindfulness and compassion. In C. K. Germer & R. D. Siegel (Eds.). *Wisdom and compassion in psychotherapy: Deepening mindfulness in clinical practice* (pp. 265–279). New York: Guilford Press.

Briere, J. (2013). Mindfulness, insight, and trauma therapy. In C. K. Germer, R. D. Siegel, & P. R. Fulton (Eds.), *Mindfulness and psychotherapy* (2nd ed.), pp. 208–224). New York: Guilford Press.

Bruce, N., Manber, R., Shapiro, S., & Constantino, M. (2010). Psychotherapist mindfulness and the psychotherapy process. *Psychotherapy Theory, Research, Practice, Training, 47*(1), 83–97.

Cambridge Insight Meditation Center. (2012). Schedule and registration. Retrieved November 25, 2012, from *www.cimc.info/schedule.html.*

Carr, L., Iacaboni, M., Dubeau, M. C., Mazziotta, J. C., & Lenzi, G. L. (2003). Neural mechanisms of empathy in humans: A relay from neural systems for imitation to limbic areas. *Proceedings of the National Academy of Sciences, USA, 100*(9), 5497–5502.

Chodron, P. (2001). *Tonglen.* Halifax, Nova Scotia: Vajradhatu.

Chodron, P. (2009). *Taking the leap: Freeing ourselves from old habits and fears.* Boston: Shambhala.

Cohen-Katz, J. E., Wiley, S., Capuano, T., Baker, D. M., Deitrick, L., & Shapiro, S. (2005). The effects of mindfulness-based stress reduction on nurse stress and burnout: A qualitative and quantitative study, part III. *Holistic Nursing Practice, 19*(2), 78–86.

Creswell, D., Way, B., Eisenberger, N., & Lieberman, M. (2007). Neural correlates of dispositional mindfulness during affect labeling. *Psychosomatic Medicine, 69*(6), 560–565.

Dalai Lama XIV. (2007, October). *Investigating the mind: Mindfulness, compassion, and the treatment of depression.* Panel discussion at Mind and Life Conference, Emory University, Atlanta, GA.

Dalai Lama XIV. (2009, May). *Meditation and psychotherapy: Cultivating compassion and wisdom.* Panel discussion at Harvard Medical School Conference, Boston, MA.

Davidson, R. J. (2004). Well-being and affective style: Neural substrates and biobehavioural correlates. *Philosophical Transactions of the Royal Society, 359,* 1395–1411.

Davidson, R. J. (2012). The neurobiology of compassion. In C. K. Germer & R. D. Siegel (Eds.), *Wisdom and compassion in psychotherapy: Deepening mindfulness in clinical practice* (pp. 111–118). New York: Guilford Press.

Duncan, B., & Miller, S. (2000). *The heroic client: Doing client-centered, outcome informed therapy.* San Francisco: Jossey-Bass.

Dunne, J. D. (2007, March). *Mindfulness & Buddhist contemplative theory.* Poster presented at the 2007 annual conference, Integrating Mindfulness-Based Approaches & Interventions into Medicine, Health Care, and Society, Worcester, MA.

Easwaran, E. (Trans.). (2007). *The Dhammapada.* Tomales, CA: Nigiri Press.

Epstein, M. (1995). *Thoughts without a thinker.* New York: Basic Books.

Epstein, M. (2008). Two person meditation: Psychotherapy with Mark Epstein. In B. Gates & W. Nisker (Eds.), *The best of inquiring mind: 25 years of dharma, drama and uncommon insight* (pp. 116–119). Boston: Wisdom.

Escuriex, B. F., & Labbé, E. E. (2011). Health care providers' mindfulness and treatment outcomes: A critical review of the research literature. *Mindfulness, 2,* 242–253.

Fain, J. (2011). *The self-compassion diet.* Boulder, CO: Sounds True.

Farb, N. A., Segal, Z. V., Mayberg, H., Bean, J., McKeon, D., Fatima, Z., et al. (2007). Attending to the present: Mindfulness meditation reveals distinct neural modes of self-reference. *Social Cognitive and Affective Neuroscience, 2*(4), 313–322.

Farb, N. A. S., Anderson, A. K., Mayberg, H., Bean, J., McKeon, D., & Segal, Z. V. (2010). Minding one's emotions: Mindfulness training alters neural expression of sadness. *Emotion, 10,* 25–33.

Feldman, C. C. (1998). *Meditation plain and simple.* London: Element.

Feldman, C. C. (2001). *The Buddhist path to simplicity: Spiritual practice for everyday life.* London: HarperCollins.

Fredrickson, B. L. (2012). Building lives of compassion and wisdom. In C. K. Germer & R. D. Siegel (Eds.), *Wisdom and compassion in psychotherapy: Deepening mindfulness in clinical practice* (pp. 48–58). New York: Guilford Press.

Freud, S. (1912). Recommendations to physicians practicing psychoanalysis. *Standard Edition, 12,* 111–120.

Freud, S. (1917). Mourning and melancholia. *Standard Edition, 14,* 237–258.

Freud, S. (1930/2005). *Civilization and its discontents.* New York: Norton.

Freud, S. (1937). *Analysis terminable and interminable. Standard Edition, 23,* 216–253.

Freud, S., & Breuer, J. (1893–1895/2000). *Studies on hysteria.* New York: Basic Books.

Fulton, P. R. (2013). Mindfulness as clinical training. In C. K. Germer, R. D. Siegel, & P. R. Fulton (Eds.), *Mindfulness and psychotherapy* (2nd ed., pp. 59–75). New York: Guilford Press.

Fulton, P. R., & Siegel, R. D. (2013). Buddhist and Western psychology: Seeking common ground. In C. K. Germer, R. D. Siegel, & P. R. Fulton (Eds.), *Mindfulness and psychotherapy* (2nd ed., pp. 36–56). New York: Guilford Press.

Galantino, M. L., Baime, M., Maguire, M., Szapary, P. O., & Farrar, J. T. (2005). Association of psychological and physiological measures of stress in health-care professionals during an 8-week mindfulness meditation program: Mindfulness in practice. *Stress and Health: Journal of the International Society for the Investigation of Stress, 21,* 255–261.

Gendlin, E. T. (1978). *Focusing* (1st ed.). New York: Everest House.

Germer, C. (2013). Mindfulness: What is it? What does it matter? In C. K. Germer, R. D. Siegel, & P. R. Fulton (Eds.), *Mindfulness and psychotherapy* (2nd ed., pp. 3–35). New York: Guilford Press.

Germer, C. K. (2009). *The mindful path to self-compassion: Freeing yourself from destructive thoughts and emotions.* New York: Guilford Press.

Germer, C. K., Siegel, R. D., & Fulton, P. R. (Eds.) (2005). *Mindfulness and psychotherapy.* New York: Guilford Press.

Germer, C. K., & Siegel, R. D. (Eds.). (2012). *Wisdom and compassion in psychotherapy: Deepening mindfulness in clinical practice.* New York: Guilford Press.

Germer, C. K., Siegel, R. D., & Fulton, P. R. (Eds.). (2013). *Mindfulness and psychotherapy* (2nd ed.). New York: Guilford Press.

Gilbert, P. (2009a). *The compassionate mind: A new approach to life's challenges.* Oakland, CA: New Harbinger Press.

Gilbert, P. (2009b). Introducing compassion-focused therapy. *Advances in Psychiatric Treatment, 15,* 199–208.

Gilbert, P. (2009c). *Overcoming depression* (3rd ed.). New York: Basic Books.

Godfrin, K. A., & van Heeringen, C. (2010). The effects of mindfulness-based cognitive therapy on recurrence of depressive episodes, mental health and quality of life: A randomized controlled study. *Behaviour Research and Therapy, 48,* 738–746.

Goldstein, J. (1993). *Insight meditation: The practice of freedom.* Boston: Shambhala.

Goldstein, J., & Kornfield, J. (1987). *Seeking the heart of wisdom: The path of insight meditation.* Boston: Shambhala.

Goodman, T. (1999, April 14). Dharma talk at Single Flower Sangha, Cambridge, MA.

Greason, P. B., & Cashwell, C. S. (2009). Mindfulness and counseling self-efficacy: The mediating role of attention and empathy. *Counselor Education and Supervision, 49,* 2–19.

Grepmair, L., Mitterlehner, F., Loew, T., Bachler, E., Rother, W., & Nickel, M. (2007). Promoting mindfulness in psychotherapists in training influences the treatment results of their patients: A randomized, double-blind, controlled study. *Psychotherapy and Psychosomatics, 76,* 332–338.

Halifax, J. (2008). *Being with dying.* Boston: Shambhala.

Halifax, J. (2012, May). *Compassion and challenges to compassion: The art of living and dying.* Paper presented at Meditation and Psychotherapy Conference, Harvard Medical School, Boston, MA.

Hanh, T. N. (1974). *Zen keys.* New York: Doubleday.

Hatcher, R. L. (2010). Alliance theory and measurement. In J. C. Muran & J. P. Barber (Eds.), *The therapeutic alliance: An evidence-based guide to practice* (pp. 7–28). New York: Guilford Press.

Hayes, S. (2004). Acceptance and commitment therapy and the new behavior therapies: Mindfulness, acceptance, and relationship. In S. C. Hayes, V. M. Follette, & M. M. Linehan (Eds.), *Mindfulness and acceptance: Expanding the cognitive-behavioral tradition* (pp. 1–29). New York: Guilford Press.

Hayes, S., & Strosahl, K. (2005). *A practical guide to acceptance and commitment therapy.* New York: Springer.

Helminski, K. E. (1992). *Living presence: A Sufi way to mindfulness & the essential self.* New York: Tarcher/Perigee.

Herman, J. L. (1992). *Trauma and recovery.* New York: Basic Books.

Hoagland, A. (2003). *What narcissism means to me.* St. Paul, MN: Greywolf Press.

Hölzel, B. K., Lazar, S. W., Gard, T., Schuman-Olivier, S., Vago, D. R., & Ott, U. (2011). How does mindfulness meditation work?: Proposing mechanisms of action from a conceptual and neural perspective. *Perspectives on Psychological Science, 6,* 537–559.

Hölzel, B. K., Ott, U., Gard, T., Hempel, H., Weygandt, M., Morgen, K., et al. (2008). Investigation of mindfulness meditation practitioners with voxel-based morphometry. *Social Cognitive and Affective Neuroscience, 3,* 55–61.

Horney, K. (1952/1998). Free associations and the use of the couch. In A. Molino (Ed.), *The couch and the tree: Dialogues in psychoanalysis and Buddhism* (35–36). New York: North Point Press.

Horvath, A., Del Re, A., Flückiger, C., & Symonds, D. (2011). Alliance in individual psychotherapy. In J. Norcross (Ed.), *Psychotherapy relationships that work* (2nd ed.). (pp. 25–69) New York: Oxford University Press.

Iacoboni, M. (2009). Imitation, empathy, and mirror neurons. *Annual Review of Psychology, 60,* 653–670.

James, W. (1890/2007). *The principles of psychology* (Vol. 1). New York: Cosimo.

Johnson, C. (2004). Reading the eightfold path. In H. G. Baldoquin (Ed.), *Dharma, color, and culture* (pp. 127–150). Berkeley, CA: Parallax Press.

Joyce, J. (1914/1991). *Dubliners.* New York: Dover.

Jung, C. G. (1938). Psychology and religion. In H. Read & G. Adler (Eds.), *Collected works of C. G. Jung 11: Psychology and religion: West and East* (2nd ed.). Princeton, NJ: Princeton University Press.

Kabat-Zinn, J. (1982). An outpatient program in behavioral medicine for chronic pain patients based on the practices of mindfulness meditation: Theoretical considerations and preliminary results. *General Hospital Psychiatry, 4*(1), 33–47.

Kabat-Zinn, J. (1990). *Full catastrophe living: Using the wisdom of your body and mind to face stress, pain and illness.* New York: Dell.

Kabat-Zinn, J. (1994). *Wherever you go there you are: Mindfulness meditation in everyday life.* New York: Hyperion.

Kabat-Zinn, J. (2003). Mindfulness-based interventions in context: Past, present, and future. *Clinical Psychology: Science and Practice, 10*(2), 144–156.

Kabat-Zinn, J., Lipworth, L., Burney, R., & Sellers, W. (1986). Four-year follow-up of a meditation-based program for self-regulation of chronic pain: Treatment outcomes and compliance. *Clinical Journal of Pain, 2*(3), 159–173.

Kabat-Zinn, J., Massion, A. O., Kristeller, J., Peterson, G., Fletcher, K., Pbert, L., et al. (1992). Effectiveness of a meditation-based stress reduction program in the treatment of anxiety disorders. *American Journal of Psychiatry, 149*(7), 936–943.

Kabat-Zinn, J., Wheeler, E., Light, T., Skillings, A., Scharf, M. S., Cropley, T. G., et al. (1998). Influence of a mindfulness meditation-based stress reduction intervention on rates of skin clearing in patients with moderate to severe psoriasis undergoing phototherapy (UVB) and photo-chemotherapy (PUVA). *Psychosomatic Medicine, 60*(5), 625–632.

Kornfield, J. (1993). *A path with heart: A guide through the perils and promises of spiritual life.* New York: Bantam.

Kornfield, J. (2000). *After the ecstasy, the laundry: How the heart grows wise on the spiritual path.* New York: Bantam.

Kornfield, J. (2008). *The wise heart: A guide to the universal teachings of Buddhist psychology.* New York: Bantam.

Kornfield, J. (2011). *Bringing home the dharma: Awakening right where you are.* Boston: Shambhala.

Kornfield, J. (2013, April 15). Holding identity lightly. Spirit Rock Meditation Center, CA. Retrieved from *www.dharmaseed.org/teacher/85.*

Koven, S. (2012, May 28). Memoirs of a slightly overweight diet doctor. *Boston Globe. www.boston.com/lifestyle/health/2012/05/27/memoirs-slightly-overweight-diet-doctor/qV19hcllxyrPPfColsedzN/story-1.html*

Kramer, G. (2007). *Insight dialogue: The interpersonal path to freedom.* Boston, MA: Shambhala.

Kristeller, J., Baer, R., & Quillian-Wolever, R. (2006). Mindfulness-based approaches to eating disorders. In R. A. Baer (Ed.), *Mindfulness-based treatment approaches* (pp. 75–91). San Diego, CA: Elsevier.

Kuyken, W., Byford, S., Taylor, R. S., Watkins, E., Holden, E., White, K., et al. (2008). Mindfulness-based cognitive therapy to prevent relapse in recurrent depression. *Journal of Consulting and Clinical Psychology, 76*(6), 966–978.

Law, N. (2008, March 31). Scientists probe meditation secrets. *BBC News Online.* Retrieved from *http://news.bbc.co.uk/2/hi/health/7319043.stm.*

Lazar, S. W. (2013). The neurobiology of mindfulness. In C. K. Germer, R. D. Siegel, & P. R. Fulton (Eds.), *Mindfulness and psychotherapy* (2nd ed., pp. 282–294). New York: Guilford Press.

Lazar, S. W., Kerr, C. E., Wasserman, R. H., Gray, J. R., Greve, D. N., Treadway, M. T., et al. (2005). Meditation experience is associated with increased cortical thickness. *NeuroReport, 16,* 1893–1897.

Levine, P. A., & Frederick, A. (1997). *Waking the tiger: Healing trauma: The innate capacity to transform overwhelming experiences.* Berkeley, CA: North Atlantic Books.

Linehan, M. M. (1993a). *Cognitive-behavioral treatment of borderline personality disorder.* New York: Guilford Press.

Linehan, M. M. (1993b). *Skills training manual for treating borderline personality disorder.* New York: Guilford Press.

Lowen, A. (1958). *The language of the body.* New York: Collier.

Lowen, A. (1994). *Bioenergetics.* New York: Penguin/Arkana.

Luborsky, L., Singer, B., & Luborsky, L. (1975). Is it true that everyone has won and all must have prizes? *Archives of General Psychology, 32,* 995–1008.

Lutz, A., Slagter, H. A., Dunne, J. D., & Davidson, R. J. (2008). Attention regulation and monitoring in meditation. *Trends in Cognitive Sciences, 12*(4), 163–169.

Ma, S. H., & Teasdale, J. D. (2004). Mindfulness-based cognitive therapy for depression: Replication and exploration of differential relapse prevention effects. *Journal of Consulting and Clinical Psychology, 72,* 31–40.

Macy, J. (2012). *The bodhisattva check-in or "My choices for this life" (current form).* Retrieved November 28, 2012, from *www.joannamacy.net/theworkthatreconnects/newpractices.html.*

Marlatt, G. A., Bowen, S., & Lustyk, M. K. (2012). Substance abuse and relapse prevention. In C. K. Germer & R. D. Siegel (Eds.), *Wisdom and compassion in psychotherapy: Deepening mindfulness in clinical practice* (pp. 221–233). New York: Guilford Press.

Marlatt, G. A., & Gordon, J. R. (Eds.). (1985). *Relapse prevention: Maintenance strategies in the treatment of addictive behavior.* New York: Guilford Press.

McKim, R. D. (2008). Rumination as a mediator of the effects of mindfulness: Mindfulness-based stress reduction (MBSR) with a heterogeneous community sample experiencing anxiety, depression, and/or chronic pain. *Dissertation Abstracts International: Section B: The Sciences and Engineering, 68,* 7673.

Michaelson, J. (2006). *God in your body: Kabbalah, mindfulness and embodied spiritual practice.* Woodstock, VT: Jewish Lights.

Miller, L. W. (2009). *Everyday dharma.* Wheaton, Il: Quest Books.

Miller, L. W. (2012, Summer). Seven month compassion series [Audio podcast]. Retrieved from *https://itunes.apple.com/us/podcast/seven-month-compassion-series/id558112558.*

Morgan, B., Morgan, S., & Germer, C. K. (2013). Cultivating attention and compassion. In C. K. Germer, R. D. Siegel, & P. R. Fulton (Eds.), *Mindfulness and psychotherapy* (2nd ed., pp. 76–93). New York: Guilford Press.

Murphy, S. (2002). *One bird, one stone.* New York: Renaissance Books.

Neff, K. D. (2011). *Self-compassion. Stop beating yourself up and leave insecurity behind.* New York: Morrow.

Neff, K. D., & Germer, C. K. (2013). A pilot study and randomized controlled trial of the mindful self-compassion program. *Journal of Clinical Psychology, 69*(1), 28–44.

Neruda, P. (1974). Keeping quiet. In *Extravagaira* (p. 26) (A. Reid, Trans.). New York: Farrar, Straus & Giroux.

Norcross, J., & Wampold, B. (2011). Evidence-based therapy relationships: Research conclusions and clinical practices. *Psychotherapy, 48*(1), 98–102.

Ogden, P., Minton, K., & Pain, C. (2006). *Trauma and the body: A sensorimotor approach to psychotherapy.* New York: W.W. Norton & Co.

Orsillo, S. M., & Roemer, L. (2011). *The mindful way through anxiety: Break free from chronic worry and redeem your life.* New York: Guilford Press.

Pennington, B. (1980). *Centering prayer.* Garden City: Doubleday.

Piaget, J. (1952). *The origins of intelligence in children.* New York: International Universities Press.

Pipe, T. B., Bortz, J. J., Dueck, A., Pendergast, D., Buchda, V., & Summers, J. (2009). Nurse leader mindfulness meditation program for stress management. *Journal of Nursing Administration, 39*(3), 130–137.

Plummer, M. (2009). The impact of therapists' personal practice of mindfulness meditation on clients' experience of received empathy (Doctoral dissertation, Massachusetts School of Professional Psychology, 2008). *Dissertation Abstracts International, 69,* 4439.

Pollak, S. M. (2013). Teaching mindfulness in therapy. In C. K. Germer, R. D. Siegel, & P. R. Fulton (Eds.), *Mindfulness and psychotherapy* (2nd ed., pp. 133–147). New York: Guilford Press.

Ramel, W., Goldin, P. R., Carmona, P. E., & McQuaid, J. R. (2004). The effects of mindfulness meditation on cognitive processes and affect in patients with past depression. *Cognitive Therapy and Research, 28,* 433–455.

Rilke, R. M. (1905/2005). *Rilke's book of hours: Love poems to God* (A. Barrows & J. Macy, Trans.). New York: Riverhead.

Roemer, L., & Orsillo, S. M. (2009). *Mindfulness and acceptance-based behavioral therapies in practice.* New York: Guilford Press.

Roemer, L., & Orsillo, S. M. (2013). Anxiety: Accepting what comes and doing what matters. In C. K. Germer, R. D. Siegel, & P. R. Fulton (Eds.), *Mindfulness and psychotherapy* (2nd ed., pp. 167–183). New York: Guilford Press.

Rogers, C. (1961). *On becoming a person.* New York: Houghton Mifflin.

Rosenberg, L. (2004). *Breath by breath: The liberating practice of insight meditation.* Boston: Shambhala.

Ryan, A., Safran, J. D., Deran, J. M., & Muran, J. C. (2012). Therapist mindfulness, alliance and treatment outcome. *Psychotherapy Research, 22*(3), 289–297.

Salzberg, S. (1995). *Lovingkindness: The revolutionary art of happiness.* Boston: Shambhala.

Salzberg, S. (1997). *A heart as wide as the world: Living with mindfulness, wisdom and compassion.* Boston: Shambhala.

Salzberg, S. (2011). *Real happiness: The power of meditation.* New York: Workman.

Salzberg, S., & Goldstein, J. (2001). *Insight meditation.* Boulder, CO: Sounds True.

Schacht, T. (1991). Can psychotherapy education advance psychotherapy integration? A view from the cognitive psychology of expertise. *Journal of Psychotherapy Integration, I,* 305–320.

Schenstrom, A., Ronnberg, S., & Bodlund, O. (2006). Mindfulness-based cognitive attitude training for primary care staff: A pilot study. *Complementary Health Practices Review, 11*(3), 144–152.

Segal, Z. V., Williams, J. M. G., & Teasdale, J. D. (2002). *Mindfulness-based cognitive therapy for depression: A new approach to preventing relapse.* New York: Guilford Press.

Segal, Z. V., Williams, J. M. G., & Teasdale, J. D. (2012). *Mindfulness-based cognitive therapy for depression* (2nd ed.). New York: Guilford Press.

Seligman, M. E. P. (1975). *Helplessness: On depression, development, and death.* A series of books in psychology. New York: Holt.

Shapiro, S. L., Astin, J. A., Bishop, S. R., & Cordova, M. (2005). Mindfulness-based stress reduction for health care professionals: Results from a randomized trial. *International Journal of Stress Management, 12*(2), 164–176.

Shapiro, S. L., & Carlson, L. E. (2009). *The art and science of mindfulness: Integrating mindfulness into psychology and the helping professions.* Washington, DC: American Psychological Association.

Sharpe, G. (2011, February 7). *The way of balance.* In Insight Meditation Society, Metta (Lovingkindness) Retreat, Barre, MA. Retrieved from *www.dharmaseed.org/teacher/75.*

Siegel, D. J. (2010a). *The mindful therapist.* New York: Norton.

Siegel, D. J. (2010b). *Mindsight: The new science of personal transformation.* New York: Bantam.

Siegel, R. D. (2010). *The mindfulness solution: Everyday practices for everyday problems.* New York: Guilford Press.

Siegel, R. D. (2012). The wise psychotherapist. In C. K. Germer & R. D. Siegel (Eds.). *Wisdom and compassion in psychotherapy: Deepening mindfulness in clinical practice* (pp. 138–153). New York: Guilford Press.

Siegel, R. D. (2013). Psychophysiological disorders. In C. K. Germer, R. D. Siegel, & P. R. Fulton (Eds.), *Mindfulness and psychotherapy* (2nd ed., pp. 184–207). New York: Guilford Press.

Siegel, R. D., & Germer, C. K. (2012). Wisdom and compassion: Two wings of a bird. In C. K. Germer & R. D. Siegel (Eds.), *Wisdom and compassion in psychotherapy: Deepening mindfulness in clinical practice* (pp. 7–34). New York: Guilford Press.

Singer, W. (2005, November). Possible biological substrates of meditation. Paper presented at the Mind and Life Institute Conference, Washington, DC.

Singh, N., Wahler, R., Adkins, A., & Myers, R. (2003). Soles of the feet: A mindfulness-based self-control intervention for aggression by an individual with mild mental-retardation and mental illness. *Research in Developmental Disabilities, 24*(3), 158–169.

Stanley, S., Reitzel, L. R., Wingate, L. R., Cukrowicz, K. C., Lima, E. N., & Joiner, T. E. (2006). Mindfulness: A primrose path for therapists using manualized treatments? *Journal of Cognitive Psychotherapy: An International Quarterly, 20*(3), 327–335.

Stiles, W. B. (2009). Responsiveness as an obstacle for psychotherapy outcome research: It's worse than you think. *Clinical Psychology: Science and Practice, 16,* 86–91.

Stratton, P. (2006). Therapist mindfulness as a predictor of client outcomes (Doctoral dissertation, Capella University, 2006). *Dissertation Abstracts International, 66,* 6296.

Surrey, J. (2005). Relational psychotherapy, relational mindfulness. In C. K. Germer, R. D. Siegel, & P. R. Fulton (Eds.), *Mindfulness and psychotherapy* (pp. 91–110). New York: Guilford Press.

Surrey, J. L., & Kramer, G. (2013). Relational mindfulness. In C. K. Germer, R. D. Siegel, & P. R. Fulton (Eds.), *Mindfulness and psychotherapy* (2nd ed., pp. 94–111). New York: Guilford Press.

Suzuki, S. (1973). *Zen mind, beginner's mind.* New York: Weatherhill.

Teasdale, J. D., Segal, Z. V., Williams, J. M. G., Ridgeway, V. A., Soulsby, J. M., & Lau, M. A. (2000). Prevention of relapse/recurrence in major depression by mindfulness-based cognitive therapy. *Journal of Consulting and Clinical Psychology, 68,* 615–623.

Teasdale, J. D., Segal, Z. V., & Williams, J. M. G. (1995). How does cognitive therapy prevent depressive relapse and why should attentional control (mindfulness training) help? *Behaviour Research and Therapy, 33,* 25–39.

Trungpa, C. (1988). *Shambhala: Sacred Path of the Warrior.* Boulder, CO: Shambhala Press.

Tryon, G. S., & Winograd, G. (2011). Goal consensus and collaboration. In J. C. Norcross (Ed.), *Psychotherapy relationships that work* (2nd ed., pp. 153–167). New York: Oxford University Press.

van der Kolk, B. A., McFarlane, A. C., & Weisaeth, L. (Eds.). (1996). *Traumatic stress: The effects of overwhelming experience on mind, body, and society.* New York: Guilford Press.

Willard, C. (2010). *Child's mind.* Berkeley, CA: Parallax Press.

Williams, J. M. G., Teasdale, J. D., Segal, Z. V., & Kabat-Zinn, J. (2007). *The mindful way through depression: Freeing yourself from chronic unhappiness.* New York: Guilford Press.

Witkiewitz, K., & Bowen, S. (2010). Depression, craving and substance use following a randomized trial of mindfulness-based relapse prevention. *Journal of Consulting and Clinical Psychology, 78,* 362–374.

Index

Page numbers followed by *f* indicate figures.

Absolute truth
  meditation as counterproductive defense
    and, 24–26
  open monitoring and, 83
  overview, 18–20
Acceptance. *See also* Nonjudgment
  compassion and, 119
  compassionate acceptance, 5–8
  overview, 2
Acceptance and commitment therapy
  (ACT), 188, 223
Acceptance-based behavior therapy for
  generalized anxiety disorder (ABBT
  for GAD), 188
Accessibility of mindfulness, 139–140.
  See also Introducing mindfulness to
  patients
Addiction, 204
Affect tolerance, 3, 48–53
Affects, moving towards the sharp points
  and, 15–16
Ambivalence, compassion and, 119
Anatta
  affect tolerance and, 50–53
  overview, 18, 20, 180
  therapeutic relationship and, 53–55
Anger, connecting with the body and,
  70–71
Anicca, 18, 20, 180

Anxiety, 165–167, 181–182
Attention. *See also* Concentration; Focused
  attention
  affect tolerance and, 48
  focused attention, 5–8
  meditation as counterproductive defense
    and, 22–23
  moving toward the sharp points and, 14
  objects of, 10–12, 11*f*
  overview, 2
Attentional control training, 12–13
Attunement, mindful therapists and, 29–30
Avoidance, 20–26
Awareness
  body awareness, 70–72, 83, 84–92,
    105–107, 150–151
  emotion awareness, 92–99
  overview, 2
  three objects of, 59–62

Balance, 120, 203. *See also* Equanimity
Beginner's mind, 55–58
Behavior, 5–8
Body
  body sensations, 16
  compassion and, 105–107
  concentration and, 70–72
  introducing mindfulness to patients,
    150–151

Body (*continued*)
open monitoring and, 83, 84–92
weaving practice into the therapy via dialogue, 152–155
Body language, 59
Body Scan, 105–107
Boundaries, professional, 191–192
Breath awareness, 72–79, 144–146
Buddha, mindful therapists and, 182–183
Buddhist meditation centers, 189–191
Buddhist psychology, 179–181

Centering prayer techniques, 12
Character issues, 157–158
Cognitive therapy, 186–187, 224
Community, mindful therapists and, 182–183
Compassion. *See also* Loving-kindness; Self-compassion
additional practices for, 202–203
ambivalence and, 119
body awareness, 105–107
concentration and, 65
eating and, 107–110
examples of treatment sequencing and, 160–174
extreme suffering and, 111–116
feeling joy for others, 129
meditation as counterproductive defense and, 25–26
overview, 100–104
sequencing practices and, 157–158
taking into daily life, 110–111
when life feels unbearable, 116–119
Compassion for the self. *See* Self-compassion
Compassionate acceptance, 5–8
Concentration. *See also* Attention; Focused attention
breath and, 72–79
connecting with the body, 70–72
equanimity and, 121
examples of treatment sequencing and, 160–174
feeling joy for others, 129
identifying the presence of, 79–81
informal practice and, 78–79
making accessible to patients, 67–79
meditation as counterproductive defense and, 20–21
moving toward the sharp points and, 15–16
overview, 5–8, 65–67, 79–81
posture and, 67
sequencing practices and, 157–158
sounds and, 67–69
therapeutic relationship and, 46
Connection, 59
Countertransference, 157–158

Counting meditations, concentration and, 80–81
Cultural factors
loving-kindness practice and, 102
mindfulness-based treatment and, 62
overview, 12–13

Daily practice, 177–178
Deathless, 176
Deeper-level meditation. *See also* Intensive practice; Practices
overview, 175–177
in the patients, 183–193
in the therapist, 177–183
Defenses, 20–26
Depression, 160–165, 205
Dharma, 182–183
Dialectical behavior therapy (DBT), 15, 188, 224
Dialogue, 151–155
Discomfort, affect tolerance and, 48–50
Discouragement, mindful therapists and, 43–44
Dissociative patients, 149
Distance, awareness and, 59
Distraction, 7, 11
"Dodo Bird hypothesis," 45–46
Dukkha, 18, 20, 180

Eating, 107–110, 188
Effectiveness of therapists, 28–29
Emotional pain, 116–119. *See also* Pain
Emotions
open monitoring and, 92–99
skills involved in mindfulness and, 7–8
Empathy, 129–131
Enlightenment, 176
Entry-level mindfulness. *See* Concentration; Dialogue; Introducing mindfulness to patients
Equanimity
additional practices for, 203
examples of treatment sequencing and, 160–174
extreme suffering and, 134–138
feeling joy for others, 129–131
forgiveness, 131–134
letting go, 136–138
overview, 120–124
sequencing practices and, 157–158
skills involved in mindfulness and, 7–8
stillness, 127–129
urge surfing, 124–127
Existential reality
equanimity and, 136–138
mindful therapists and, 181
Expectations, realistic. *See* Realistic expectations
Experiential focus, 16–18

Faith traditions, 12–13. *See also* Religious
  practices
Fear, loving-kindness practice and, 111
Feelings
  awareness and, 59
  concentration and, 66–67
  moving toward the sharp points and,
    14, 15–16
  open monitoring and, 83
Flow of relationship, 59. *See also*
  Therapeutic relationship
Focused attention, 5–8, 14, 46–48, 65–67.
  See also Attention; Concentration
Forgiveness, equanimity and, 131–134
Formal practice. *See also* Practices;
  Sequencing practices
  for the clinical day, 37–41
  maintaining, 33–34
  mindful therapists and, 30–31, 31–
    35
  overview, 8–10
  posture for, 34–35
  weaving practice into the therapy via
    dialogue, 151–155

Goal of treatment, 175–177
Gratitude, 25–26
Grief, 19
Group mindfulness programs, 185–186

Homework, assigning additional practice
  as, 64

Identity construction, 54–55
Images
  moving toward the sharp points and,
    14, 15–16
  open monitoring and, 6
Impermanence, 18, 20, 180
Impulses, 5–8, 15–16
Individualized practice, 4–20, 11f, 17f,
  20–26. *See also* Practices
Informal practice. *See also* Practices;
  Sequencing practices
  for the clinical day, 41–43
  concentration and, 78–79
  mindful therapists and, 30–31
  overview, 8–10
  weaving practice into the therapy via
    dialogue, 151–155
Inpatient settings, introducing mindfulness
  to patients, 149
Insight, equanimity and, 121
Intensive practice. *See also* Deeper-level
  meditation
  meditation as counterproductive
    defense and, 22
  meditation centers, 189–191
  mindful therapists and, 30–31

patients and, 189–190
  resources regarding, 216–223
Intention, formal practice and, 34
Interpersonal attunement, 58–59
Interpersonal conflict, compassion and,
  114–116
Intrapersonal attunement, 58–59
Introducing mindfulness to patients
  fragile or vulnerable personalities and,
    148–151
  how to start, 140–148
  overview, 139–140
  weaving practice into the therapy via
    dialogue, 151–155

Joy, equanimity and, 129–131
Just listening stance, therapeutic
  relationship and, 48

Kindness, 146–148. *See also* Loving-
  kindness

Labeling, emotion awareness and,
  94–97
Listening
  additional practices for, 204–205
  concentration and, 67–69
Loss
  equanimity and, 134–138
  loving-kindness practice and, 103–104
  relative or absolute truth and, 19
Loving-kindness. *See also* Compassion
  additional practices for, 205–206, 208
  ambivalence and, 119
  concentration and, 65
  examples of treatment sequencing and,
    160–174
  extreme suffering and, 111–116
  introducing mindfulness to patients,
    146–148
  meditation as counterproductive defense
    and, 25–26
  overview, 100–104
  phrases for cultivating, 102
  safety and, 14–15
  sequencing practices and, 157–158
  skills involved in mindfulness and, 7–8
  taking into daily life, 110–111
  when life feels unbearable, 116–119

Meditation centers, 189–191, 216–223
Meditation in general, 20–26, 213–216
Memories
  moving toward the sharp points and,
    15–16
  skills involved in mindfulness and, 7–8
Metta (Pali term). *See* Loving-kindness
Mindful self-compassion (MSC), 105,
  187–188

Mindful therapist. *See also* Therapist
    consultation and, 35–43
    deepening therapeutic presence, 46–53
    deeper-level meditation and, 177–183
    feeling discouraged, 43–44
    formal meditation instruction and
        practice and, 31–35
    forms of practice and, 30–31
    overview, 26–30, 44
Mindfulness overview, 1–2, 2–3, 3*f*, 213–
    216. *See also* Introducing mindfulness
    to patients
Mindfulness-based cognitive therapy
    (MBCT), 186–187, 224
Mindfulness-based eating awareness
    training (MB-EAT), 188, 224
Mindfulness-based psychotherapy
    deeper-level meditation and, 185–192
    overview, 3, 26
    resources regarding, 223–224
    roles of mindfulness, 3*f*
    sequencing practices and, 156–158
    transitioning to, 62–64
Mindfulness-based relapse prevention
    (MBRP), 187
Mindfulness-based stress reduction
    (MBSR), 184, 186, 189, 223
Mindfulness-building techniques, 14–15
Mindfulness-informed psychotherapy, 3, 3*f*
Mistakes, loving-kindness practice and,
    104
Moving toward the sharp points
    equanimity and, 133
    meditation as counterproductive defense
        and, 24
    overview, 13–16, 17*f*
Multitasking, avoiding, 36–37

Narcissistic preoccupations, therapeutic
    relationship and, 53–55
Narrative focus, 16–18, 76–78
Nirvana, 176
Nonjudgment, 2. *See also* Acceptance
No-self, 50–55, 180. *See also Anatta*
Not knowing, therapeutic relationship and,
    55–58

Open monitoring
    body awareness and, 84–92
    concentration and, 65
    emotion awareness and, 92–99
    equanimity and, 121
    examples of treatment sequencing and,
        160–174
    feeling joy for others, 129
    moving toward the sharp points and,
        15–16
    not knowing and, 56
    overview, 5–8, 82–84, 97–99

sequencing practices and, 157–158
Open space, therapeutic relationship and,
    48
Openness, equanimity and, 121

Pain
    additional practices for, 208
    compassion and, 116–119
    open monitoring and, 90–92
    resources regarding, 224
Patient variables
    deeper-level meditation and, 183–193
    introducing mindfulness to patients,
        148–151
    meeting patients where they are and,
        158–160
    sequencing practices and, 156–158,
        160–174
Pausing, 37, 151. *See also* Slowing down
Personas, therapeutic relationship and,
    54–55
Perspective, equanimity and, 120–121,
    122, 134–136
Physical pain, 116–119. *See also* Pain
Posture for meditation, 34–35, 67
Practices. *See also* Formal practice;
        Informal practice; Intensive practice
    Accepting the Challenge meditation,
        134–135
    All Things Must Pass meditation,
        136–137
    Anchor at the Bottom of a Stormy Sea,
        127–128
    Answering the Phone meditation, 43
    Awareness of Emotions in the Body
        meditation, 92–93
    Awareness of Sensation meditation,
        89–90
    Beginner's Mind meditation, 57
    Being Present meditation, 140–142
    Being with Discomfort meditation,
        49–50
    Body Sweep meditation, 87–88
    Breathing Together exercise, 60–62
    Bringing Compassion into Daily Life
        meditation, 110
    Compassion in the Moment meditation,
        202–203
    Compassionate Being meditation, 112,
        113, 167
    Compassionate Body Scan meditation,
        105–106, 162, 166
    Compassionate Eating meditation,
        108–109
    Connecting With the Suffering of Others
        meditation, 117–118
    Cradling the Breath meditation,
        76
    Dialogue Meditation, 154–155

Embracing Emotions that Arise in Therapy meditation, 51–52
examples of treatment sequencing and, 160–174
Feeling Three Breaths meditation, 144–145
Finding Our Professional Shadow exercise, 54–55
Finding the Breath meditation, 73, 161
Finding the Pattern meditation, 97–98
Flash Cards, 211
Forgiveness: Letting Go of Poison meditation, 132–133
Four-Elements Meditation, 203
Hands meditation, 204
Labeling Emotions meditation, 94–95, 113, 137, 163, 169, 172
Letting Go of the Story meditation, 77–78
Listening to Another meditation, 204–205
Lotus Growing in a Murky Pond, 205
Loving-Kindness for Clinicians meditation, 205–206
Meditation with Light, 206
Merging with the Source meditation, 38
Mind That Sparkles meditation, 207
Mindful Meal Breaks meditation, 42–43
Mindful Termination: An Account of the Journey activity, 173–174
Mini-Mindfulness Break meditation, 39
Mountain meditation, 122–124, 170
No-Show meditation, 40–41
Not Worrying About Me meditation, 53–54
Offering Loving-Kindness to Oneself meditation, 103
Opening to Kindness meditation, 146–147
Returning to the Anchor meditation, 42
Riding the Wave meditation, 125–126, 187
Seeing with Loving Eyes meditation, 208
selecting, 195–211
Shelter in Place meditation, 210–211
Silly Walking meditation, 208–209
Simply Listening meditation, 68, 85, 161, 168–169
Soles of the Feet meditation, 209
Standing Meditation, 142–143
Sympathetic Joy meditation, 129–130
Thoughts Are Only Passing By meditation, 209–210
Three Objects of Awareness meditation, 59
tonglen, 116–117, 151, 172
Touch Points meditation, 70, 106–107, 113, 166, 168, 204

Walking in the World meditation, 207–208
Walking Meditation: Anchoring in the Body, 84–85, 164, 166, 168
Walking to the Waiting Room meditation, 31, 41
What Brings You Away? meditation, 47–48
Working with a Difficult Person meditation, 114–115
Presence, 29–30, 46–53
Professional boundaries, 191–192
Psychiatric disorders, introducing mindfulness to patients, 148–151
Psychotherapy
meditation as counterproductive defense and, 20–26
narrative and experiential focus and, 16
relative or absolute truth and, 19–20
roles of mindfulness, 3*f*
Psychotic patients, introducing mindfulness to patients, 149

Realistic expectations, concentration and, 79
Reenactments, sequencing practices and, 158
Refuge, mindful therapists and, 182–183
Relational mindfulness, therapeutic relationship and, 58–62
Relationships, compassion and, 114–116
Relative truth, 18–20, 24–26
Religious practices
loving-kindness practice and, 102
meditation as counterproductive defense and, 23–24
mindfulness-based treatment and, 62
overview, 12–13
Remembering, 2
Resonance, mindful therapists and, 29–30
Restraint, affect tolerance and, 49–50
Retreat practice
meditation as counterproductive defense and, 21–22
mindful therapists and, 32, 178–179
overview, 8–10

Sacred pause, 37. *See also* Slowing down
Safety, 13–16, 17*f*, 24
Sangha, mindful therapists and, 182–183
Sati (Pali term), 2
Secular practices
loving-kindness practice and, 102
meditation as counterproductive defense and, 23–24
mindfulness-based treatment and, 62
overview, 12–13

Self-compassion. *See also* Compassion
    equanimity and, 124
    safety and, 14–15
    skills involved in mindfulness and, 7–8
Self-criticism, skills involved in mindfulness
        and, 7–8
Self-esteem, relative or absolute truth and,
        19
Sensations, awareness and, 59
Sensory experiences, open monitoring
        and, 6
Sequencing practices. *See also* Formal
        practice; Informal practice
    examples of, 160–174
    meeting patients where they are and,
        158–160
    overview, 156–158, 160–174
Shadow, therapeutic relationship and,
        54–55
Simplicity, mindful therapists and, 36
Single-mindedness, mindful therapists and,
        36–37
Skills involved in mindfulness, 5–8
Sleeping problems, connecting with the
        body and, 71–72
Slowing down, mindful therapists and,
        36, 37
Sounds, concentration and, 67–69
Spaciousness, mindful therapists and, 36
Spiritual bypasses, 24–25
Stillness, equanimity and, 127–129
Suffering
    affect tolerance and, 48
    breath and, 76–78
    compassion and, 111–116
    equanimity and, 123–124
    loving-kindness practice and, 103–104
    open monitoring and, 6, 82–84
    therapeutic relationship and, 59–62
Suicidal impulses, sequencing practices
        and, 158

Termination, examples of treatment
        sequencing and, 171–174
Therapeutic process, mindful therapists
        and, 29–30
Therapeutic relationship
    deepening therapeutic presence, 46–53
    letting go of narcissistic preoccupations,
        53–55
    mindfulness training and, 28–29
    mindfulness-based treatment and, 62–64
    moving toward the sharp points and,
        15
    not knowing and, 55–58

    overview, 45–46
    relational mindfulness, 58–62
    relative or absolute truth and, 19–20
    sequencing practices and, 157–158
Therapist. *See also* Mindful therapist
    deeper-level meditation and, 177–183
    effectiveness of, 28–29
    goal of treatment and, 177
    introducing mindfulness to patients,
        140–148
    meditation as counterproductive defense
        and, 20–26
    mindfulness training and, 27–30
    mindfulness-based treatment and, 62–
        64
    overview, 27–28
    professional boundaries and, 191–192
    professional shadow and, 54–55
    relative or absolute truth and, 19–20
    roles of mindfulness, 2–3, 3f
Thoughts
    awareness and, 59
    concentration and, 66–67
    moving toward the sharp points and, 14
    open monitoring and, 6, 83
Tonglen
    additional practices for, 202–203
    examples of treatment sequencing and,
        172
    introducing mindfulness to patients, 151
    overview, 116–117, 191
Transference, sequencing practices and,
        157–158
Trauma, 167–171, 210–211
Truth
    meditation as counterproductive defense
        and, 24–26
    open monitoring and, 83
    relative or absolute truth, 18–20

Unconditioned, 176
Unsatisfactoriness, 18, 20, 180
Urge surfing, 124–127, 187

Vipassana, 190
Vulnerabilities, sequencing practices and,
        157–158

W.A.I.T. acronym (Why Am I Talking?),
        therapeutic relationship and, 57–58
Words, awareness and, 59

Zen centers, 190–191, 216–223
Zone of tolerance, introducing mindfulness
        to patients, 151